A Country Doctor Writes:
CONDITIONS
Diseases and Other Life Circumstances
Hans Duvefelt, MD

Published by
A Country Doctor Writes, LLC
acountrydoctorwrites.com

A Country Doctor Writes:

CONDITIONS

Diseases and Other Life Circumstances

Hans Duvefelt, MD

PREFACE

The 100 stories and vignettes in this book are about some of the diseases and circumstances that affected patients I have come across in my more than 40 years in medicine.

All of them were originally posted on my blog, "A Country Doctor Writes", which I published for a dozen years, a project with a total word count somewhere over 350,0000 - like "Moby Dick" and "For Whom the Bell Tolls" combined, although I am not making any direct literary comparisons.

As a non-native English speaker I give much thought to words that even though they look and sound similar don't exactly correspond to words I first learned in Swedish, my mother tongue.

The English word "condition" is such a weighty word. It covers both medical and non-medical challenges we face as human beings, in expressions like "name a condition associated with visual hallucinations of elf-like characters" and, obviously, "suffering is part of the human condition".

The less imposing Swedish word "kondition" is merely used to describe what shape something is in, like "as new" or "fit".

So, in this little volume I am thinking like a true American, mixing diagnoses I have made, missed or just come across with some of the human circumstances and destinies, tragedies and victories that I have been privileged to witness.

1) AN OLD, NEW DIAGNOSIS

The middle aged woman started to pull down her jeans as she explained:

"I want you to look at this rash on my leg. I've had it for a month now."

What I saw got my mind churning. On top of her left thigh was a brown discoloration about the size of the palm of my hand. It had a reticular pattern, like a coarse lace doily or irregular fish net. It was light brown, smooth to the touch and didn't blanch when I pressed on it.

I knew I had read something about rashes that looked like that, but I couldn't remember any details. So I did what I often do, I googled the description:

(Images) Brown reticular erythema.

Almost instantly I saw a perfect picture of the woman's rash. The caption read "Erythema ab igne".

Yes, that was it, but what was it again?

My trusted Wikipedia had a tidy little entry that echoed with memories in the recesses of my mind. I printed it out for her. It described the rash as often occurring in older patients who used hot water bottles or, in the old days, stood too close to the fire to keep warm.

I didn't think my patient slept with a hot water bottle only on her left thigh.

"Is anything warm often touching that spot?" I asked.

"Yeah, my laptop", she answered instantly.

"Try putting a folded towel or something between your leg and your laptop", I said as we wrapped up her visit.

What an odd symmetry, I thought to myself: A diagnosis of historical interest, brought back by the use of modern technology and identified by the very device that causes it.

2) MORBUS PROPEDEUTICUS

It was spring. My medical school class, two years along in our five-and-a-half year endeavor, had earned the "medicine kandidat" degree. We were now worthy of leaving the basic sciences and research center on the outskirts of town and starting our preparatory clinical, "propedeutic" semester at the University Hospital. In Sweden, at that time, we used a lot of Latin words and phrases. Crohn's disease was Morbus Crohn, chart notes listed physical exam findings by Latin names for the bodily organs: Cor for the heart, Pulm(ones) for the lungs, Hepar for the liver, etc.

Uppsala Academic Hospital was an imposing campus, with several tall, white towers, housing the most modern wards, laboratories and operating theaters. We were relegated to a pink stucco building that housed the old tuberculosis clinic.

The physical exam course was taught by a couple of older pulmonologists. At first they struck many of us as relics from a bygone era, but as the course went on, our respect grew. These unassuming physicians could percuss a patient's chest wall and describe in detail what the x-ray would look like, they made us feel the tip of the spleen by turning the patient on his right side, they measured jugular venous pulsations and pedal pulses.

Sometimes we had real patients with remarkably abnormal findings to examine, but we often were charged with examining each other for assessment of normal physical exam findings.

My partner for the Lymphatic System module was Sven Björk, a slow-talking kid from the very north of Sweden. He had jet black, completely straight hair and a broad face with eyes set wide apart. He was part Same, the native, reindeer-herding nomadic population from north of the Arctic Circle.

Sven was a bright young man. He had memorized the anatomy quicker than I had, well ahead of the exercise. Yet he seemed nervous. I soon found out why: He had noticed several enlarged submandibular and anterior cervical glands on himself. We compared each other's necks and jaw lines, but found to our surprise that our lymph nodes were about the same size.

My glands had been big as long as I could remember; I had gone through repeated strep infections. In second grade I missed 42 days in just one semester. Sven had never had strep throat, and he didn't remember feeling any enlarged lymph nodes before, but he had also never checked himself quite like this before.

Our instructor came over to see how we were doing. Sven cleared his throat and started telling Doctor Bruun what both Sven and I had noticed on his neck.

The fifty-something doctor put his hands on Sven's neck. Methodically, he worked his way up, down and around the neck and down into the armpits. He had Sven lie down on the exam table, supine for the liver, on his right side for the spleen, then reached for the lymph nodes in Sven's groin. His face was serious as he whisked Sven off to his office, leaving me standing, feeling my own cervical lymph nodes, bigger than Sven's.

Sven was diagnosed with Hodgkin's Disease, a type of lymphoma that wasn't quite as easily cured then as it is now, but Sven responded well to the treatment and didn't miss much school.

The rest of our class, me included, went through a prolonged case of what our instructors called Morbus Propedeuticus, Medical Student's Disease. It is natural to worry that you might have some of the bad diseases you learn about in medical school. Seeing one of your classmates develop cancer sets the stage for more than the normal amount of hypochondriasis.

I realized that even though Sven's and my lymph nodes were similar, his had developed quickly without reasonable explanation and mine had been there for years and had their origin in my recurrent episodes of tonsillitis. I did ask my instructor to check me over, which he gracefully did. He was not worried, and I accepted his assessment. I never again worried about having a dreadful disease, but I often thought of Sven and me during that physical exam class; there but for the grace of God go I.

Around the time of my birthday a couple of weeks ago, I suddenly thought of Sven again: I know he was declared cured from his Hodgkin's, but what about freak recurrences, late cancer treatment effects or other tricks of the Grim Reaper?

Google gave me the answer: Sven is head internal medicine physician at a medium sized hospital. He has published several scientific articles, and was interviewed recently about differences in heart attack survival between northern and southern Sweden. I even found a couple of pictures. Wouldn't you know it, he doesn't have a gray hair on his head or wrinkle in his face; he looks younger than I do.

Bless you, Sven. I wonder if you know how often my thoughts have gone back to those weeks we spent together way back then.

3) CLINICAL PNEUMONIA OR VIRTUAL HEALTH?

"So, are you saying Bobby really didn't have pneumonia?" Mrs. Halstead asked. Her eleven-year-old son, a boy with multiple medical problems, had been in the office ten days before with fever, a bad cough, right-sided chest pain with each deep breath, and very loud crackles in the lower portion of his right lung. His blood count was normal and his chest x-ray looked almost normal - you could argue that it looked a little streaky in the right lower lobe, but the city radiologist who read his x-ray without actually listening to his lungs thought it was a normal set of pictures.

Bobby felt good at his follow-up appointment, and his lungs sounded clear. So, had I been wrong in diagnosing him with pneumonia when the radiologist didn't agree with my interpretation of the films?

I remembered the case of Fanny Brown, my receptionist's mother. She had a nasty cough and was losing weight. Her chest x-ray was normal, but her CT scan showed a tumor the size of a baseball - we all know a chest x-ray isn't always the final word on what is wrong with a patient.

I tried to explain to Mrs. Halstead that a camera, even one used for x-rays, has its limitations.

"If you see a pretty rainbow and pull out your camera to capture it, but the picture doesn't show the rainbow, does that mean you didn't see a rainbow?" I tried.

There is an old Swedish military and Boy Scout joke, which I heard in both places: When the map and the terrain disagree, you go by the map in the military and by the terrain in the Boy Scouts. I spent more time as a Boy Scout than as a soldier - my inclination has always been to trust my assessment of the terrain.

I was on call for Christmas, and had a few days off around New Year's. Catching up on my journals, I was delighted to find a piece in the December 25th edition of The New England Journal of Medicine by Abraham Verghese, MD, entitled "Culture Shock - Patient as Icon, Icon as Patient". Dr. Verghese describes teaching residents, who seem more inclined to look at their patients through the "eyes" of the electronic medical record than through bedside clinical observation. He also talks about what to do when the map and terrain don't seem to agree. He quotes Alfred Korzybski, the Polish-American philosopher credited with founding the theory of general semantics, who said, "the Map is not the Territory". I'm not sure which of the two Korzybski thought was more real.

Bobby Halstead had been ill, and now he was well. I don't know what his mother really thought of my diagnosis of his pneumonia, but it was a great illustration of what Dr. Verghese wrote about a short while later in "The Journal": *Our technology, invented as a way to document clinical reality, has almost become more real than the disease states it was designed to document.*

4) VISIONS OF LITTLE PEOPLE

Richard Westman was a fine-boned, soft-spoken eighty year old retired accountant, who prided himself of his sharp intellect and excellent memory. I had known him for a few years, but didn't see him often as he was relatively healthy. Then a myocardial infarction robbed him of his physical stamina, and he started to develop heart failure. He also developed heart rhythm problems, and ended up with a pacemaker and on a blood thinner. We saw a lot of each other during the last two years of his life - or I saw more of him than he saw of me, as he suffered from advancing macular degeneration.

He was familiar enough with our office layout that a casual observer might not have noticed how visually impaired he was. He needed help managing his medication bottles, and he had long before lost his ability to read and watch television. He listened to books on tape, and he followed the news with great interest; there was nothing wrong with his mind, or so I thought.

Then one day he confided in me that he saw things - children, sometimes groups of them, playing in the yard outside his kitchen window in broad daylight. They always seemed friendly and happy, never threatening. They never spoke, never made a mess and never pulled any pranks.

At first he was unnerved by seeing them, but gradually he came to enjoy their presence. He confided in me:

"I don't really think they are there, but I don't know why I see them."

"Do you want them to go away?" I asked.

"No, they just puzzle me" was his answer.

I had at first thought of offering him a trial of a mild antipsychotic, but it was clear that he didn't need that, since the visions didn't frighten him in any way.

We talked about the children now and then, but I soon forgot about his visions. Then one day his wife called the office and said their daughter had found something on the Internet they wanted me to read. The had figured out that Mr. Westman suffered from Charles Bonnet Syndrome, CBS.

Most of the time it isn't a thrill when patients or their families bring in articles they have found online. We all know that more information is not the same as better information. But this time I was fascinated by what they brought to my attention, and I soon found myself digging deeper into the subject on my own:

First described in 1760 by a Swiss philosopher, who noticed that his grandfather, who was almost blind, saw birds and other figures that weren't there, Charles Bonnet Syndrome (CBS) typically affects older people with severe vision loss. CBS often only exists for a year or two as vision deteriorates, and can involve geometric patterns or little creatures, often elf-like, usually friendly looking and often with hats. The visions are rarely threatening and they are common - at least 10% of people with worse than 20/60 vision are said to have this syndrome.

CBS is not a psychological condition. It is believed to be something similar to phantom pains, where a person even after an amputation can "feel" a missing extremity, even though they know perfectly well that it isn't there. The visual cortex of our brains is always "filling in the blanks" when we look at something quickly or when we cannot see things quite clearly. Any type of visual impairment, such as cataracts, diabetic retinopathy or macular degeneration, can create more "blanks", which are automatically "filled in" by the brain. Antipsychotics don't seem to be of any help.

Some writers like to think of Charles Bonnet Syndrome as a portal to paranormal experiences or parallel universes. For me it was a portal to being more willing to see what patients and their families drag into the office after surfing around the Internet!

5) OFF THE RECORD

Gwen and Dan Olsen were a handsome couple with a stunning blonde eight-year-old daughter, Trina. They had just moved to the town where I did my residency and over the course of their first six months there I saw all three of them for routine health care needs.

One day Gwen came in for nausea. She didn't look well and I could see in her facial expression that something was dreadfully wrong. Thinking unplanned pregnancy and morning sickness, I glanced at her problem list, where her husband's vasectomy was listed, in my own handwriting, as her method of contraception.

"I'm pregnant", she burst out, tears suddenly streaming down her cheeks.

I sat quietly for a while. She didn't say anything.

"Dan had a ...", I started.

"He's not the father", Gwen said.

Wiping her tears she described how she had gone back to her parents for a visit, run into an old boyfriend and found herself doing the unthinkable.

"Does Dan know?" I asked.

She nodded.

"What do you want to do?" I didn't say the A-word, but she understood.

"We've talked it over and we're going through with the pregnancy as if it were Dan's baby", she began. "He's promised me he will love us both just as much as if he were the father. We'll just tell people the vasectomy must have failed."

"Those things happen", I said.

"Will you be my doctor for the pregnancy?" she asked.

"Of course", I nodded.

"And please don't put anything in my medical record about it not being Dan's."

"Of course", I reassured her.

That fall I delivered a beautiful baby boy to two of the nicest, proudest parents I know. I was able to see him, his parents and his sister through two years of well baby visits, shots and minor childhood illnesses during the last two years of my residency.

Several years later I happened to run into the four Olsens again. Little Brad looked just like his mother.

Today I read in a journal that a large percentage of patients won't tell their doctor sensitive information if they believe their information might be shared electronically with other doctors, hospitals or insurance companies.

Some things are better left off the record.

6) A TRAIN WRECK WITH TWO CAR WRECKS

Carlos Sanchez was lucky to have survived the accident. His almost brand new car was totaled, and he was taken to the hospital, strapped on a rigid back board with a cervical collar. No fractures were found; he was sore all over, and didn't remember much of the accident, but it was the first snowstorm of the winter and it was assumed he had driven too fast for the road conditions and simply lost control of his car. I signed the copy of his emergency room report and his chart went back to our clinic's medical records room.

One week later, Carlos' chart was on my desk again. This time, he totaled his rental car, and again he escaped serious injury. What an unusual thing to happen, I thought. Carlos seemed like such a slow-moving, sensitive young man; why would he be out crashing cars every week? I signed off on his report, and his chart went back to be filed again.

The next day was Friday and I was looking forward to my weekend off. My wife and I were planning a trip to town for some Christmas shopping and a late dinner at our favorite restaurant.

Just before five o'clock, Carlos showed up at the front desk and said, "I just don't feel good".

I took one look at him, and agreed with his assessment; he just wasn't right. He had some sort of encephalopathy, that was clear, and he had an unusual pale, yellow coloring. My wife came to join me, and we headed up to town, with Carlos willingly in the back seat. We swung by the emergency room, dropped him off with a few words exchanged with the clinician on duty.

The final diagnosis was acute kidney failure; he was admitted, underwent emergency dialysis, and some time later received a kidney transplant. Last year he rejected his new kidney, so he is back on dialysis, waiting for another kidney.

The moral of the story is that even car accidents during the first snowstorm of the season may happen for a reason, and when someone has two car wrecks in a short period of time, the onus is on the treating physician to ask why.

7) CHILDREN WHO NEVER GREW

I have two patients with phenylketonuria. Both are about my age. Laura, a non-verbal, slender woman with weathered features but the mind of a very young child, lives in the community. Her sister, Regina, has lived all her life in a nursing home. She doesn't have a wrinkle in her face, and seems mostly unaware of her surroundings.

The two girls were born several years before Dr. Robert Guthrie developed the blood test for phenylketonuria, and a decade before routine PKU screening was introduced in this country. I often wonder what the parents of these two girls knew about their condition, where they went for a diagnosis, and if they even got one while Laura and Regina were still young. In many cases back then, PKU went undiagnosed as the specific cause of mental retardation.

Pulitzer and Nobel Prize winning author Pearl S. Buck gave birth to a daughter, Carol, in 1921. Carol did not develop normally, and on the advice of her Chinese doctors, Pearl Buck traveled to the Mayo Clinic to have her evaluated. She left the clinic and the United States without a diagnosis, except "I don't know. Somewhere along the way, before birth or after, growth stopped".

Pearl Buck cared for Carol at home until age nine. At that point she returned to America. She wrote "The Good Earth", her book about her experiences in China, in 1931 with the hope of making enough money to support her daughter, who was institutionalized around that time. In 1950, she wrote "The Child Who Never Grew" a memoir about her daughter. It wasn't until ten years later that the cause of Carol's mental retardation was finally diagnosed as phenylketonuria, the genetic disease that wasn't even known until Carol was in her early teens.

The disease had first been described in Norway twenty years before Laura and Regina were born. Its discovery involved another set of siblings:

Dr. Asbjørn Følling, who had been a chemist before studying medicine, was asked to evaluate a brother and sister with severe mental retardation. His son, Ivar, told the story in a speech (http://www.pkunews.org/about/history.htm) on the sixty year anniversary of this event in 1994:

"The stage is set in 1934. A mother with two severely mentally retarded children came to see my father, and to ask for his advice...She had also noticed that a peculiar smell always clung to her children...

The girl, 6.5 years old, could say a few words, was fond of music, had a spastic gait and a whimsy way of moving about, apparently at random. At times she had an enormous appetite, at other times none. The boy, almost 4 years old, could not speak or walk, eat or drink on his own. He was unable to fix his eyes on anything, and stool and urine habits were those of a baby."

Dr. Følling's son went on to describe his father's painstaking chemical analyses of the children's urine over the next several months that led to the realization that they both excreted phenylpyruvic acid, which healthy individuals don't. The disease, phenylketonuria, is still called Følling's disease in Norway.

The diet necessary for PKU patients was slowly established once Dr. Følling's chemical analyses of urine hinted at their abnormal breakdown of the essential amino acid phenylalanine. An infant formula was developed in 1951. There are now protein supplements with low levels of phenylalanine, and also a pill that lowers phenylalanine levels, Kuvan (sapropterin), developed in the last decade.

Laura comes to see me every three to four months. I see her sister, Regina, every week during my nursing home rounds.

When I see her, I always think about the life changing benefits of the newborn PKU test that came about in my own lifetime.

Laura and Regina are part of the history of medicine, some of the last few with a cruel disease few doctors today have ever seen. I feel sad and humbled in the presence of these two contemporaries of mine, two children who never grew, but I also feel inspired by the steady progress of basic science.

8) ALTERED VISION

Sweden, Saturday night:

Sitting in my aunt's living room on the eleventh floor as the late summer sun set and the sky turned dark, the conversation over after-dinner-coffee and cognac turned to her recent stroke and emergency carotid artery surgery. My mother had a small stroke a couple of years ago, which fortunately only affected her peripheral vision to her right. My aunt's sequelae are less specific, affecting a few fingers, her balance and some parts of her memory. I let my gaze wander to my right from the coffee table to her windowsill with several blooming orchids and the city lights below.

"How funny", I thought to myself, "there's a spider web between those two orchids".

A perfect, round spider web sat between the two orchids with a distant light source illuminating it from behind. I tilted my head to make sure; my aunt was always a good housekeeper and it seemed unlikely she would have cobwebs on her orchids. "Maybe the stroke did even more things to her", I thought to myself.

With my head tilted I saw another spider web of the exact same size and appearance, between the next two orchids on the windowsill, also illuminated by a bright light in the distance. "No way she would have two cobwebs", I decided. "It must be my eyes".

As the conversation continued I drifted off with my own project. Closing one eye at a time and discretely tilting and turning my head, I determined the spider webs were only visible with my right eye. Sudden cataract of one eye seemed an unlikely diagnosis, so I figured it must be something else, probably a vitreous detachment. I saw no flashing lights, which can be a symptom of either a vitreous or a retinal detachment, and there certainly was no curtain over any part of my visual field or any loss of peripheral vision.

With no ominous diagnosis immediately apparent to me, and not wanting to ruin the evening, I beamed myself back to the conversation and finished out the evening without saying a word about my vision.

Driving back to the hotel, I knew for the first time what people mean when they describe the difficulties of night driving with cataracts. The spider webs seemed more like small haloes around streetlights and headlights of oncoming cars. This is a classic symptom of cataracts, but this was too sudden. Squinting with my right eye allowed me to drive comfortably.

After parking the car outside the hotel I continued my exploration. What looked like a halo with a spider web configuration was also a circle filled with a swirl of movement, like water circling a drain. Inside this swirl of water were squiggly, small worm-like shapes, similar to the small, unobtrusive floaters I have had for years.

I went up to my room and pondered my fate. I wanted to be a doctor from about the age of four, ever since as a sickly child I had our general practitioner come for house calls. When I became severely and progressively nearsighted starting at age seven, I became fascinated with ophthalmology. My first eye doctor was a thin, old man with an office in an ancient apartment building with marble stairs, oak doors and a musty smell. As he leaned into me with his bright lights, he spoke with great concern about my worsening eyes. Every year I would get new, thicker lenses, and every year he would seem more concerned. After puberty, things seemed to slow down, and the old doctor seemed to be more content with my situation. He was so wise and kind. I wanted to be just like him.

In medical school I flirted with the idea of becoming an ophthalmologist; I learned everything I could about refraction, and as an avid photographer and dark room enthusiast, it seemed like a natural fit. I took electives in ophthalmology and thought this would be my life's work.

Then one thought, one factoid, stopped me in my tracks: As a severe myopic, I might be at increased risk for suffering a retinal detachment - then where would I be as an eye doctor who couldn't see well? The rest, as they say, is history. I decided to become the kind of general practitioner I first identified with as a young child.

Fast forward to 2008, a middle aged Family Practitioner, sitting in a hotel room with a self-diagnosis of a vitreous detachment in a country where I no longer have any medical connections - do I have a harmless condition with no need for intervention? Do I trust what I think I know about ophthalmology beyond my own specialty training? Do I trust whoever is on duty at the small hospital nearby? Or do I call my wife back home in the States and ask her to pull some strings and get me an appointment Wednesday with the best ophthalmologist I know back home?

9) ORTHOREXIA NERVOSA - TOO MUCH OF A GOOD THING

In Swedish, there is a word that just can't be translated succinctly into English. "Lagom" means "just enough" or "adequate", but it is saturated with overtones of moderation, contentedness and political, even social, correctness.

"Lagom" is a way of life - moderation in everything. It is no surprise that Swedish newspapers seem to be on the lookout for stories about people who stray from that middle-of-the-road way of life. One story in Dagens Nyheter caught my eye (for interested/concerned readers, my right eye is almost back to normal) during the flight back to the States this morning. It sent me out on the Internet once I landed and got connected to the airport wireless network:

"Exaggerated Healthfulness Can Lead to Serious Disease" is a feature about a 30-year old woman, who after eating a lot of junk food while living in the US started on a journey filled with strict diets and rigorous exercise. She never thought she was too fat, which is the defining feature of Anorexia Nervosa, but she somehow felt she had to eat extremely healthfully to compensate for her prior indiscretions. Her condition, Orthorexia Nervosa (obsession with healthy eating), described by Steven Bratman in 1997, although not officially recognized, is getting increasing attention. Its complications are not dissimilar from those of Anorexia Nervosa, as it can lead to malnutrition with all its consequences.

I had not run into the term before - figures I would run into it in Sweden, the Mecca of Moderation. I can see that this is a culture-dependent variety of Anorexia Nervosa, which was first described in the late 1800's as Fasting Girls. The culture was not focused on healthfulness the same way then as it is today. In Victorian times, fasting was of body image and spiritual interest, and Fasting Girls were said to have mystical powers.

Our current DSM-IV (Diagnostic and Statistical Manual of Mental Disorders) classification of Anorexia Nervosa doesn't mention restricting foods based on their healthfulness, and Orthorexia Nervosa isn't recognized in it at all. I looked around for blogs on the topic, and found some, including "There's no such thing as orthorexia nervosa, it's only a fancy term for a health food junkie". I like that title, because I think that whenever there is a "new" disease or when an "old" disease gets more attention, patients tend to over-report the symptoms of it and doctors have a tendency to over-diagnose it. While the DSM-IV has weight criteria that help keep the diagnosis of Anorexia Nervosa more objective, most psychiatric diagnoses hinge on value-laden words like often, intense or undue, which are all subjective to some degree.

I have said before that there is a tendency (at least in the US) to medicalize the human experience. The last thing we want to do is start calling "health food junkies" sick; let's not forget that "junk food junkies" have been well proven to get very bad complications from their food choices, too!

I have made the observation a few times that the spectrum of what we call the human experience can be defined by what lies at the extremes or by the nuances within the range where most people find themselves.

People say "I'm depressed" even if they know they are only experiencing a temporary sadness. They say "I have OCD", even if they don't meet the DSM-IV criteria.

Going too far with our words isn't always the most effective way to communicate. Now that there is a new medical term with no DSM-IV definition behind it yet, we all need to be careful how we use it. Let "health food junkies" be just that as long as they don't suffer medical or social consequences. Let's restrict use of the new medical term for people who, as Steven Bratman originally suggested, suffer negative consequences of their behavior.

It is ironic that we now have a new disease for people who do everything they can think of to be healthy.

This is where the concept of "lagom" comes in: Instead of holding perfect eating and maximum exercise as an ideal, we should all do as the Swedes, and aim for pretty good eating and pretty adequate exercise.

I guess it's always hard to see for yourself when you cross the line to extremism. As the old Swedish saying goes: "Lagom är bäst!"

10) A RARE FORM OF DEAFNESS OR A TRIVIAL CASE OF CONGESTION?

I chose doxycycline to treat Norman Starks Lyme disease. A week later he went to a walk-in clinic with sudden loss of hearing in his right ear. The PA who saw him suspected that the doxycycline had caused it and told him to stop the medication. Meanwhile, he needed at least one or two more weeks of antibiotics. He got amoxicillin.

When I saw Norman I asked what kind of exam they had done on him, he said "they just looked in my ears".

"Did they do any kind of hearing test?" I asked.

He shook his head.

"Did they put a tuning fork on your head?"

"No", he said quizzically.

I pulled my tuning fork from a plastic basket on the counter. I have one in every room.

"So how is your hearing now?" I asked.

"I think it's a little better."

"OK, tell me, if I put this tuning fork in the middle of your head like this, where do you hear it the loudest?"

Norman looked like he concentrated hard. He seemed confused.

"It's louder in my right ear."

"And which of these is louder, on the bone behind your ear or in the air in front of it?"

"Behind."

I put the tuning fork away and sat down next to him.

"Your hearing is going to be fine. You can hurry it along by using some cortisone nose spray for a while. This is not nerve deafness, you're just congested. And the doxycycline had nothing to do with it."

I love low tech medicine

And just the other day I saw a new diabetic who complained of blurry vision. After a split second of worry, I excused myself and got several sheets of dark paper, stapled them together and pierced a small hole in the center.

"Come with me, let's check your vision", I said.

We went down the hall and I asked him to look at the eye chart through the pinhole, one eye at a time.

"What's the smallest line you can read?"

"D,E,F,P,O,T,E,C", he read.

"Perfect. The lenses inside your eyes are just swollen from your high blood sugars. Hold off a little before seeing the eye doctor, and don't order glasses until your blood sugars have settled down."

Another early lesson all the way back from medical school.

11) A LOUSY DIAGNOSTICIAN

The tall, youthful seventy year old woman wore her strikingly white hair in a tight bun. She was dressed like a Donald Fagen song - in jeans and pearls ("Maxine", 1982).

She had an intense burning, itching sensation on the left side of her neck and occiput. Looking closely at her neck and hairline, I saw a couple of small, red papules. A few of them looked like early blisters.

I suspected herpes zoster and offered her a generic antiviral. The earlier you start it, the better your chances of avoiding long lasting pain afterward, I explained.

A week later, there were some red blotches and several scratch marks. Her burning and itching were worse.

I prescribed gabapentin and told her how to titrate herself up from 100 mg at bedtime to 300 mg three times a day.

The following week she still had red blotches and scratch marks and felt no better. I frowned.

She said "My granddaughters have head lice, so I asked my daughter to check me, but she couldn't find any. Would you check me, just to make sure?"

I leaned close and removed my -11 diopter glasses. My focal point is about one finger length from my corneas.

It took me a while, but I found half a dozen nits, enough to be sure she had the real thing.

Didn't I feel a little sheepish. Seventy year old woman with burning and itching scalp? Must be zoster, right? Head lice is more of a pediatric problem, right?

Wrong. I narrowed my differential diagnosis too quickly.

And, I didn't take my glasses off the first time.

12) THE DANCE

The band members brought their instruments and their small amplifier system into the activity room through the big glass doors facing the parking lot. As they tuned their instruments and warmed up, the residents started to stream into the big, bare room.

Some arrived in their hospital beds, some were pushed in their wheelchairs, some shuffled in with canes and walkers and a few strolled in unaided with the spring of anticipation in their steps.

There had been bands there before, but this was a real dance band with horns, percussion and a female vocalist.

He walked down the long hall with a group of others from the dementia unit. By now he knew the way, even though his eyes failed to guide him because of his advanced macular degeneration. He could see the nurse's aides in their brightly colored scrubs, but he had trouble making out his fellow residents in the slow caravan.

As they approached the activity room he heard the sweet sound of the vocalist and the wind instruments. The rhythm energized him and he remembered dancing to Glenn Miller and Artie Shaw tunes like "In the Mood" and "Begin the Beguine" in the Forties. He suddenly felt sad. Where was his wife? Why wasn't she there with him?

One of the aides escorted him to a chair along the sidewall, close to the band. They were playing something Latin he didn't know what to dance to. He couldn't see if anybody was dancing yet, but the music was cheerful and made him feel good.

Eyes turned toward her as she entered the room. She felt pretty in her blue dress and shoulder-length black hair. She saw him sitting by the band and quickened her steps, her left leg swinging outward in a slight semicircle and her arm kinked at the elbow. It had been six months since her stroke and this was her first dance since then.

He noticed the blue dress as she approached him, but couldn't tell at first who she was.

"Have you been waiting long?" she asked.

"Well, hello, dear. I just got here."

"I'm so glad to see you", she whispered in his ear before planting a discreet kiss on his cheek. She sat down next to him. She made sure to place herself so she could touch him with her good arm.

The band started playing a new song. He realized after the first few bars that it was "Tuxedo Junction". Years ago he would have done the Lindy Hop to it, but he couldn't pull that off now. This would be a nice, slow swing dance.

"May I have this dance?" he asked.

"Well, certainly", she answered and gave him a slight squeeze.

She led him onto the improvised dance floor with her right arm and they stood there for a few bars, her right hand in his left, both of them just moving slightly to the rhythm. He led her into first the basic step, then a push-out and then an underarm turn. She followed beautifully. They danced the whole song without saying anything at all.

The next tune was a slow waltz. She was able to put her left arm up on his right one and he danced gently with small steps. His eyes strained to see her facial expression, but he didn't see the tears that had begun to well up in the corners of her eyes.

"I'm sorry I was away for such a long time", she whispered.

"It's all right", he answered, patting her on the back as they danced.

"I was really sick and couldn't come to see you."

"It's okay."

He didn't see all the little scars on her bare arms or the tracheostomy scar over her windpipe.

"I'm so glad I am here with you today."

"I'm glad you came", he said and added "I love you."

By now, two floods of tears were streaming along her pale cheeks and down her neck, across her demon and snake tattoos, wetting her jet-black hair.

"I love you too, Grandpa."

13) LOSING A PATIENT TWICE

I had some down time this past weekend and spent some of it looking at what Swedish physicians are writing in their blogs. I came across a little piece by a 25-year-old Swedish resident, who connected with a patient on her ward in his fifties (her father's age), who seemed to be doing OK, but died overnight while she was off duty.

I tried to remember the first patient I lost, but I couldn't. There have been so many in all my years as a doctor, some lost prematurely, but most in their old age and after a long illness.

A few months ago, a former patient who no longer lived in our town, died. He was only a few years older than my own children and the news of his death affected me deeply, even though I hadn't seen him for years.

Bobby Smith was a normal, rambunctious, ten year-old until one day, my second winter in town, when we got a radio call from the ambulance. In those days we had all volunteer EMT's, and none had any advanced training, so the doctors at our clinic would get called to go on ambulance runs.

It had snowed heavily that morning and school was cancelled. By noon the snowfall had stopped, and the sun came out. Bobby went sledding right in front of his house. At first, the new powder slowed him down, but every time Bobby followed the same path down the hill he went faster and farther. The last time, he ended up in the middle of the road.

Samuel Trumbull, the town selectman, didn't have a chance to avoid hitting Bobby as he lay on his sled in the middle of the road.

The ambulance had twenty miles to go on the winding, slippery road to the hospital. Bobby was unconscious, not breathing, but with a good pulse and blood pressure. I maintained his airway and bagged him the whole way.

He pulled through, but with severe brain damage. He never spoke again. He would make grimaces and smile or poke at you. He was bed bound and incontinent. I did house calls there for a few years. Eventually they wheeled him into his old classroom, mainstreaming him, as they called it.

His parents split up, and Bobby ended up moving away from town. I would still often think of Bobby, and poor selectman Trumbull - his life was never the same after that day, either.

Suddenly, one day this spring, a patient whose maiden name was Smith - something I never reflected on - cancelled an appointment because her brother had died. When I saw her a week later, she mentioned who her brother was. All of a sudden I was back in that ambulance, bagging this little boy, who could have been my own son. I lost Bobby all over again, but this time I lost him forever.

14) NORMAL BLOOD PRESSURE

Dwight Frost had all the risk factors, plus he had already had a stroke several years ago. His blood sugars were too high, his lipid profile was near the top of the class, he still smoked a cigar now and then, and his blood pressure hovered around 200. He also seemed a little vague about which medications he actually took and which ones he didn't.

He spoke rapidly with a slight tremulousness in his voice and seemed to be eager for the visit to be over.

On his second visit he brought a big bag of medications, not just the neatly written list his wife had sent him in with the first time. Some of the bottles were marked on the lid "AM" or "PM", others said "BP", "sugar" and some had a rubber band around them, which seemed to mean he was definitely taking them as prescribed.

His thyroid function and other routine labs were normal. At both visits I recorded his blood pressure in both arms; I had him sit and stand; the first time I saw him, I also checked the pressure in his right leg.

His wife was a retired nurse, he told me, and she also checked her own blood pressure with a stethoscope and a manual sphygmomanometer. She had recorded almost daily blood pressures, all under 140, that she had done on him between his two visits with me. She couldn't come in with him, because she was actually bedridden from severe arthritis. She rarely got out of the house to see her rheumatologist, the only doctor she had.

I thought for a moment. There was only one way I could resolve this, so I asked:

"Would you mind if I stopped in next Friday afternoon to check your blood pressure when you're relaxing at home?"

"Anytime, were always home", he answered.

Friday afternoon I drove across town in a light snowfall. The faint February sun filtered its way between the snowflakes, which seemed to sparkle and rotate in the air ahead of me without ever hitting the windshield.

The Frost home was a tidy ranch house with an ell connecting it to the garage. Dwight saw me drive up and greeted me at the door.

Ada, his wife, was lying on a day bed near a pellet stove in the paneled room. A large Persian cat was sleeping at her feet.

Dwight walked over to a Canadian rocker near his wife's bed and sat down. As we made small talk, the majestic cat woke up and moved over to Dwight's lap. Slowly, almost absentmindedly, Dwight patted the cat and told me she was almost twenty years old.

I noticed that Dwight spoke without the tremor in his voice I had heard at the office, and he exuded a calm that I had not seen in him before.

As I watched from the chair he had offered me, a slow ritual unfolded before me. With the cat in his lap, Dwight placed the blood pressure cuff on his arm and gave the stethoscope to his wife. "Ready", he said to Ada, and when she nodded, he pumped the cuff up and then slowly deflated it.

"134/82", she said.

I walked over, put my own cuff on his arm instead and pulled out my own stethoscope from the pocket of my tweed jacket.

As I pumped up the cuff, Dwight patted his cat, who started purring, and leaned his head back against the back of his chair.

Slowly deflating the cuff from a high of 240, I listened in anticipation. At exactly 132, I heard the first Korotkoff sound. I continued to deflate the cuff and finally had my answer.

"Your blood pressure is fine", I said, and reached down to record the numbers. "It's just high when you come in to the office. So, why don't you come and see me in three months, and just bring your readings from home."

I gathered my equipment. As I looked up again, Ada and Dwight were holding hands. He was not the same anxious man I had seen in the office twice before. The cat was still in his lap, sleeping.

15) TWO CASES OF BUBBLY URINE

I saw two patients with a chief complaint of bubbles in their urine this month.

One middle aged woman had eaten some wild mushrooms she was pretty sure she had identified correctly, but once her urine turned bubbly a few days later, she came in to make sure her kidneys were okay.

Even though she was feeling quite well they were not and she ended up going straight to Cityside hospital for IV fluids, a kidney biopsy and dialysis. We don't know yet how much her kidney function will recover and we still don't know if the mushrooms had anything to do with it.

I saw her in followup the other day and she was taking everything in stride, showing more curiosity than fear and despair.

The other, a generally healthy woman, came in for sudden swelling of her ankles. She mentioned her urine had been bubbly for months. She had googled her symptoms and was convinced she had either acute kidney or heart failure. She felt weak.

Her review of systems had several positives, including joint pain. Specifically, one knee had been swollen and painful for a while.

"Have you taken any ibuprofen or naproxen for your knee?" I asked.

"Yes, why?"

"Nonsteroidals can cause sodium and fluid retention", I explained.

Her cardiovascular exam was normal.

Because of her obvious anxiety, I minimized the EMR on my computer screen and googled "leg edema NSAIDs" and showed her that Dr. Google agreed with me that this was a plausible explanation.

"The problem with Google is that it displays possible diagnoses without ranking their probability. Exotic things may rank higher because more people look them up", I explained.

She understood but was visibly not reassured. She did agree to hold the ibuprofen for a while to see if her swelling resolved and to get some labwork to check her kidney function.

So far, I know that her kidney function is perfectly normal. We'll see if her swelling goes away and stays away.

I didn't tell her that I once had a woman about her age come in one December day with just a little ankle swelling and, ten years later, ended up with a heart transplant.

As I told another patient the other day, it is my job and not the patient's to think of the worst case scenarios.

16) A CHANGE OF HEART

It was the day before Christmas 1996, and Betsy Billings was not the type to run to the doctor unnecessarily. She had been unusually busy since Thanksgiving, trying to get ready for Christmas, and the virus she had come down with in November seemed to have left her with a profound sense of fatigue.

For a few days she had noticed ankle swelling, which brought her to the office on Christmas Eve.

Betsy had always been a bright, cheerful woman, who seemed to take everything in stride. She spoke in a high-pitched, youthful voice at age 50, had a contagious smile that included a peculiar way of squinting, and she had the funniest way of acting out what she talked about, almost like playing charades.

Her leg edema was significant, and there was deep pitting that persisted after I removed my fingers. Her neck veins were a little distended, and her heart was enlarged on her chest x-ray. She admitted to sleeping on two pillows because of shortness of breath when lying flat, and she had put on weight.

I started her on fluid pills that day and ordered an echocardiogram. Her EKG didn't look like she'd had a heart attack.

That day was the beginning of a long journey for Betsy, who almost to the day ten years later had to rush to Boston when her pager went off in the middle of the night because a donor heart was available.

During the ten years between her diagnosis of cardiomyopathy and her heart transplant she required more and more tinkering with her medications. She was my first patient on carvedilol, a beta-blocker specifically introduced for use in heart failure. When I was in medical school, beta-blockers were contraindicated in heart failure. When carvedilol was first introduced, patients had to be kept in the office to be monitored for dropping blood pressure after their first dose.

In the beginning of Betsy's journey, I had to double check things with our local cardiologists, and as time went along, my backup shifted to her transplant team in Boston.

The transplant happened quicker than we had expected, because of the availability of a perfect donor match. During the next several months I didn't see Betsy at all; I just got the reports from Boston.

When I first saw her after her surgery she was on high-dose prednisone and all kinds of immunosuppressants to prevent rejection. It was a strange experience. She was a changed woman. She was physically changed from the steroids, and she had none of her usual cheerfulness and optimism. She doubted she could ever lose the weight she had gained, and she suffered from anxiety I had never seen in her before.

The obvious explanation was the steroids; I have seen before how steroids can change a person's psychological makeup. But in Betsy's situation, I couldn't help but wonder what it does to a human being to have another person's heart beating in their chest. I don't know that all of our personality is located in our brain, with all the talk about cellular memory and other such things we hear about today.

During Betsy's first year of living with a new heart, and while on steroids, she struggled less successfully than before with her weight issues. She had a minor spending spree on one of the TV shopping networks, and her husband, Robbie, was sometimes perplexed by her moods. She even asked to be referred to a psychiatrist.

Last month I saw her again, and she looked great. She was on a low dose of prednisone, needed almost no heart medications, and mostly came to see me for a flu shot and some routine lab tests. She told me about her August vacation trip, when she had rented a bicycle and for the first time since she got sick gone on a bicycle picnic with her sister.

As she spoke, tears streamed down her cheeks, and her funny little squint was back. She made little body movements like charades again, and I saw the Betsy I had known before her transplant. She's a new woman in a way, but also back to her old self.

17) INVISIBLE TIES

Kirk Donner has been my patient for eighteen years, ever since his adoptive parents brought him home at age two weeks. He is their pride and joy, very wise for his years, talented in languages and sports and strikingly handsome. He is taller than his parents with olive skin, curly dark hair and brown eyes, contrasting with their fair complexions and reddish blond hair.

He had known he was adopted from early on. At his well-child visits he would explain to me that he didn't grow in his mother's belly but in her heart as she longed for a baby to love some day.

His parents told him his birth mother was very young and wasn't able to take care of him. She placed him for adoption because she wanted the best for him, they had explained.

Kirk often wondered what she was like and if they had a lot in common. His adoptive parents knew very little about her. They had a medical history questionnaire and a short biographical sketch from the adoption agency. They knew her first name was Suann.

A few times in moments of anger he had lashed out at his parents: "You don't love me! I wish I could live with my real mother", but most of the time he was happy with his life and didn't even think about being adopted.

For several years before his eighteenth birthday the Donners had promised to take him to the State Capital if he wanted to go to the adoption registry. He knew that by registering there, he might be able to find his birth mother.

Kirk hesitated. He was very curious about her, but he also worried about what it would be like to meet her. Would she be someone he could respect and how would she feel about him? His eighteenth birthday passed and he still wasn't sure.

Then a classmate's mother had a car accident and was nearly killed when a moose ran into the road in front of her car. Kirk decided to make the trip as soon as possible.

With his adoptive mother he decided on a day and they made a date of it with lunch at a nice restaurant across the street from the registry. Kirk enjoyed the food but didn't eat with his usual appetite. They had agreed that he would go alone while Beth Donner had coffee and they would meet back at the car when he was done.

Kirk took the elevator to the fourth floor. He was alone. As the door slid open, he stepped forward and almost collided with a tall, dark-haired woman with designer jeans and a plain, white blouse. Her eyes met his as he stopped and apologized. They were large and kind. She flashed a smile as he swerved around her, embarrassed and eager to get to the registry.

He walked up to the receptionist and stated his errand with words he had practiced in his mind the whole trip.

The clerk handed him a form and as he reached for a pen he saw a stack of similar forms in front of her. Reading the top one upside-down he saw the name:

Suann Walker.

18) "I HATE COMING HERE"

It's another Monday morning at the substance abuse clinic. It is my turn as the doctor in the black swivel chair in the corner office overlooking a half-vacant strip mall.

Today's first inductee is a pregnant 22-year old with track marks on her forearms. Her obstetrician and caseworker at the Department of Human Services made her come. It is obvious she is less than thrilled.

"How long have you been doing opiates", I ask with my fingers hovering over the keyboard. She tells her story, first in monosyllabic monotone, but as we move through the questions and she realizes I am not there to lecture her on anything, she warms up a little.

Because she is pregnant, she didn't arrive here in withdrawal out of concern for the fetus. Her last use was the night before. I explain how to place the Subutex tablets under the tongue and avoid swallowing, so the medication is fully absorbed through the mucous membranes of her mouth. Then I fill out the prior authorization form for Medicaid. I make sure to put her due date on the form, so she will be approved until she delivers. Then I write the prescription, sign it and spell out my name and my special DEA number for opiate replacement prescriptions.

My next inductee is in a cold sweat. He is the same age as my own son. He snorted some Oxys and Ritalins Friday night. Today he has the shakes and the runs. He has no job, is in trouble with the law, and he has been here before, but was discharged because of repeated failed urine drug screens.

I document his COWS score, the degree of physical withdrawal he is in. He had been doing high doses, so I prescribe him 16 mg of Suboxone daily. I explain that since last time he was here, we have switched from tablets to strips that melt under your tongue the same way. He knows; he knows everything about opiates. Is he here again because of his circumstances, I wonder, more than from a deep desire to quit right now? His counselor's notes in the computer record have a hint of skepticism in them.

"I hate coming here", says my third patient for the morning. He is a foreman at a nearby factory, logging week number 178 in the program. He is on 2 mg per day. Going from 3 to 2 mg, he had a terrible time with both physical symptoms and cravings.

"I wish I didn't have to be on this stuff. I want to be over this. I sit in the waiting room with these people who trade stories about what they have done, and I don't want to hear it. I have a job, a family, and I hate having to come here for my lousy prescription, but I know I can't keep my life together without it."

Fourth up is a woman in her forties I haven't seen before. She transferred in a week ago when Dr. Feiner sat in this chair. I recognize the woman's name. She is a physician, who just lost her license a few months ago. She is stable on her dose. I write the prescription and she leaves quietly.

The next patient is a mother of two, who just had surgery for ovarian cancer. She is in obvious pain. We had talked last time about how Suboxone does help with pain, but it is not all that potent. She had told me then that she was more afraid of falling back into addiction than being in pain.

This time, she is tearful. Her cancer has already metastasized, and she speaks of what will happen to her two girls if she can't be cured. She winces with pain, and I ask her again if she is sure she wants to stay in the program. Her husband already manages the Suboxone strips for her, and he could manage pain medications for her as well. But she knows that the naloxone in her Suboxone strips keeps her from feeling the same high that other opiates give.

"I am so grateful for what this program has done for me, that I don't want to risk that, even for this", she says and points to her abdomen. "Whatever time I have left.." She chokes, tears streaming down her cheeks, and blows her nose with tissue from the box on the corner of my desk. "Whatever time I have left, I want to be sober, and I want to be all there for my girls and for my husband. I don't want to be strung out."

"I hear you", I say. But you are in pain, I can see that." She nods.

"I'm going to increase your dose back up to our maximum. That will make some difference. But you may be helped by something like a fentanyl patch, that stays on for three days at a time..."

"Thanks, but this is fine", she says as she takes her new prescription and strains to rise from the visitors' chair by the window.

I rise and open the door for her. Then I close it and sit down quietly in my black swivel chair for a few minutes as I look out over the boarded-up windows of the empty storefronts across the parking lot.

I don't hate coming here, as some of the patients do. It is sobering to think back on the ones who are forced to come here, the ones who come here when they can't afford their drugs of choice, the ones who fight valiantly to get their lives back in order and the ones who have lost, or are about to lose, everything.

19) A WORK EXCUSE

Bibi and Dwight, both in their mid-sixties, always move as a unit. They have been married for forty years. Early on, they were athletic and adventurous, but over the past five or six years Dwight has developed macular degeneration and a fairly severe case of arthritis.

I have seen him once a year for a physical and usually no more. At his last two physicals, Bibi brought up her concern that Dwight was tired. She has always been present for his visits, even before his eyesight started to fail him. He always downplayed his fatigue and blamed it on his age.

This time I focused my exam on different causes for fatigue and ordered several blood tests. Bibi seemed pleased, but Dwight seemed distant and unengaged. I suspected he might be depressed about his arthritis and near blindness. We agreed to have a follow-up to go over the test results.

The only remarkable thing about his results was a borderline low thyroid function, which usually doesn't cause any symptoms at that level.

As it happened, Bibi had her own appointment with one of my colleagues at the same time as Dwight came back to go over his test results.

After greeting him, I started:

"Well, Dwight, all your blood work looks fine..."

"I was sure it would", he interrupted. "Listen, Doc, I know why I'm tired", he said with a tone of frustration in his voice.

"I love Bibi, but she's not like you or me", he began whispering. "From the crack of dawn till way past anybody's normal bedtime, we have to work. In the spring and summer it's the

47

gardens. We grow more vegetables than we could possibly eat. In the fall it's the raking and the firewood. We are three years ahead on wood now. In the winter we dust and reorganize all her books and knickknacks. We never relax; we never sit down and talk. She always has to be busy. She's wearing me out, Doc!"

He raised his arms in a gesture of exasperation.

"Help me, Doc!"

Just then, there was a knock on the exam room door. Autumn, my nurse, peeked in and said:

"I've got Bibi here, are you ready for her to join you?"

I glanced at Dwight. His eyes sank to the floor as he nodded.

"So, how is my boy?" Bibi said as she sat down next to Dwight while I quickly gathered my thoughts.

"Well, it's nothing serious", I said, "but Dwight has subclinical hypothyroidism, which is due to an autoimmune process in the thyroid. Some people get quite tired with that, more than you might expect from the thyroid numbers alone. Coupled with his arthritis, I expect Dwight to be more tired both physically and mentally than he was a few years ago."

Both Bibi and Dwight had their eyes on me as I came to my concluding statement:

"I think with more rest built into his day, he should be good for many more years."

As we said good-bye, his knotted hand squeezed mine quite hard for a person with arthritis.

20) WRESTLING THE ROOSTER

"I used to be strong, I wrestled the bull", Sumner Ball said, "but now I can't even wrestle the rooster".

On the far side of eighty years old, he looked lively and trim, and his weathered face hinted at a smile as his blue eyes peered straight into mine.

"I think these cholesterol pills are hurting my muscles", he declared. "I don't think they're good for me".

"Is it your back?"

I scanned through his last few visits and saw he had mentioned some low back pain while gardening this summer.

"No, Dr. Tom took care of my back", Sumner said, referring to our local chiropractor. "My arms and my legs hurt, even my shoulders hurt."

Years ago, Sumner had developed polymyalgia rheumatica, and it took almost two years to get him through it with the help of gradually decreasing steroid doses.

"Let me get a blood test, and why don't you stop the cholesterol pills for a while and see how you feel", I offered. We agreed to have a follow-up visit in a few weeks.

Three weeks later, Sumner Ball was a changed man. His faint smile was now a big grin.

"I knew that medicine was not good for me. I feel better now, not so many muscle aches. And I stopped the other one too. It was making me dizzy."

"What about the blood thinner?" I asked.

"No, that one I take. I know it can keep me from having a stroke. But I know my body, and I know what my body needs, just like when I had goats and horses - they knew what to eat and not to eat."

"My goats don't always know the difference", I said. Sumner grinned as he continued, "and we didn't have the vet come out all the time. We treated them with herbs, good feed and common sense."

His blood pressure was still OK, but his pulse rate was just under 100, a little high for someone with atrial fibrillation.

"Your diltiazem was keeping your heart from going too fast", I reminded him.

"I feel good now. I like to stay this way. Do you think I am making a mistake?" His penetrating, small blue eyes told me he didn't want me to disagree with him.

"Your heart could start racing", I warned him. "Let me see you in a few weeks to make sure you're not going into heart failure."

Two weeks later, Sumner had gained five pounds. His legs were swollen, he was short winded and his irregular pulse was 130.

"Your heart is missing the diltiazem", I said.

"I can't take it", Sumner answered. I knew he had already tried a beta blocker a few years ago, and his pulse had dropped to 40 on the lowest dose.

"How about trying something natural?"

His eyebrows rose. I continued: "There is an old herbal remedy, made from foxglove, called digitalis. It may slow your heart down enough to get you out of trouble."

A week later, Sumner looked like he'd take on something much bigger than the rooster again. His pulse was 80 and his weight was back to its baseline. Leaning back in his chair, he said:

"The third day I took your medicine, I could feel my heart slow down. I knew that herb medicine would be good. You do all right by me."

"I figured something more natural might work for you", I answered. "Besides, it was the only other thing I could think of."

"I like you. You have common sense", he said as he offered me his large hand.

It was the firm handshake of a man who had worked hard all his life.

21) OFF COURSE

"Elsa Bruegger has seemed a little unsteady in the morning lately", the charge nurse told me at my boarding home rounds two weeks ago. "Her morning blood sugars have been a little low. Do you think we should cut back on her insulin?"

"Sounds reasonable", I answered. Let me look at her chart." Elsa is on valproic acid as a mood stabilizer and sees her psychiatrist every three months. Her drug level was just about due to be checked, so I ordered a fresh set of labwork and decreased the dose of her long-acting insulin.

We continued our stand-up rounds, going through dozens of reports and issues on the many residents who were not scheduled to be seen that day. I then did two admissions and saw a couple of patients for their scheduled visits.

The next time I went to the boarding home, I checked on the results of Elsa's blood tests and reviewed her blood sugar log. Everything was well within range.

"How is she doing?" I asked.

"The girls still find her a little off balance now and then, especially in the morning."

"Tell me again how long this has been going on..."

"Probably a month or a month and a half."

"Any urinary symptoms? Anything else going on?" I flipped through the chart again. My eyes fell on some insurance paperwork. There, two months ago was a rejection letter for a Prior Authorization request for a brand-name drug Elsa had been taking for urinary frequency.

"Well, she's incontinent sometimes, but that's not new, and she has no dysuria. But we did have to switch her to that generic drug for her urine two months ago", the charge nurse answered.

"Well, if she's still incontinent, let's stop the pill, because that could cause her to be dizzy", I said, "so let me write the order for that."

Yesterday I stopped in at the boarding home again to speak with the family of one of my patients. While standing at the nurses' station I happened to see Elsa coming down the hall with her walker.

With every step Elsa took, she and the walker veered more and more to the right until she came to a stop with the right front wheel against the wall. She then lifted the walker toward the middle of the corridor and started walking again. Eight or ten steps later, she was back against the wall. She stopped and lifted the aluminum walker toward the middle of the corridor again and repeated the same procedure.

"Look", I whispered to the nurse.

We watched as Elsa repeated her zigzag veer and correction half a dozen times until she came to the TV room half way down the hall. After she settled into her chair, I asked to borrow her walker. She seemed bemused.

I picked it up and spun the wheels, which rolled without any apparent resistance. I checked the length of its four legs and the tightness of all its bolts.

"Let me just take it for a spin", I said. Elsa grinned as I started walking.

The moment I put even the slightest pressure over the front wheels, the walker started turning towards my right. I hit the wall just as fast as Elsa had. She giggled. The nurse sighed with her hands on her hips.

"Let's get you a new walker!" I said as I returned the defective unit to Elsa. She smiled and nodded.

I didn't know whether to feel good or bad about my diagnosis. It had taken more than two weeks, but really only took a minute to arrive at once I got on the right course.

22) AN AMENDED DIAGNOSIS

I must admit I had felt a little smug about my discovery of Elsa Bruegger's faulty walker. It really seemed like a very logical explanation to her walking into walls all the time. As it happened, her new walker didn't quite solve the problem. She continued to be off balance and sometimes did seem a bit unfocused, even downright sedated.

Looking back through her record, I came across a mildly elevated ammonia level a few months ago. I remember speaking with her psychiatrist back then about Elsa and a couple of other patients we share, whose routine ammonia levels were mildly elevated. Elsa had a standing order from the psychiatrist for ammonia levels every three months because of her valproic acid (Depakote) prescription for her mood disorder.

All my research has led me to the conclusion that ammonia levels are of little or no value in predicting whether patients on valproic acid are headed for trouble due to the drug's unpredictable tendency to cause ammonia to build up within the central nervous system. I have come to understand that ammonia levels are only slightly helpful even in assessing a patient with coma or near coma; the correlation between brain levels and peripheral blood levels of the toxic ammonia relate poorly to each other because of how the blood-brain barrier works to keep the chemistries inside and outside the central nervous system separate. Many experts recommend against routine measurements of ammonia levels for this reason.

Watching Elsa fumble her way down the hall, I decided to order an ammonia level "just in case". It came back elevated - twice as high as it had been ten weeks ago. Her liver function tests were normal.

I ordered her valproic acid stopped and made sure her psychiatrist got a copy of the lab report and my notes.

This week, Elsa is finally walking straight. She is attending her day program, says "good morning", makes good eye contact and smiles. She also shows more of a temper, but nothing inappropriate.

Maybe this time I finally got it right.

23) A RED HERRING

When Joel Mulholland fell off his garage roof last winter he must have hit every bone in his upper body. The muscular, tattoo-armed, motorcycle-riding fifty-five-year old, who had never complained of pain or even taken a sick day before, became almost unable to work.

His x-rays at the emergency room showed no fractures and his blood tests during our office follow-ups showed no evidence of any inflammatory disease. Our local rheumatologist, Norm Fahler, saw him several times and made a diagnosis of cervical myofascial syndrome. I followed Joel for his cholesterol medication. The blood tests showed no sign of muscle damage from the medication. I even asked him not to take the pills for a month to make sure they weren't causing his muscle and joint pain.

The muscle relaxant and nonsteroidal medications offered him some relief, but the physical therapy did not. Joel was discouraged. He had a brand new Harley-Davidson motorcycle sitting in his new garage, and he told me he was beginning to wonder if he would be able to ride it when spring came.

Joel's neck seemed to get slowly better. He had full range of motion and not as much tenderness as before, but his shoulders were in constant pain and his range of motion was not improving.

He had some heartburn, so I gave him an acid blocker, concerned that his arthritis medication might be putting him at risk for an ulcer. That took care of his indigestion, but soon thereafter Joel's appetite started to dwindle. We did some blood tests again and I made a follow-up appointment for the following week.

The day after our appointment Joel's wife called. This was unusual; he never let anyone else speak for him. She reported that he was nauseous and had vomited twice that morning. I called in some nausea medication and advised Sandy to bring him to the hospital if the vomiting wasn't controlled with the medication.

That weekend felt like the first day of spring. The sun was bright, the roads were dry, and there were motorcycles in town and on the County road. I kept thinking of Joel and his new Harley-Davidson. What was wrong with him?

Monday morning's faxes from the hospital brought the answer: Joel was admitted for intractable vomiting. His blood tests were normal, except for some signs of dehydration. His scans showed a normal looking liver, pancreas and gallbladder, but there was a little fluid at the bottom of his right lung and in the upper lobe there was a large tumor that had not been visible on plain x-rays.

I copied the hospital reports to the rheumatologist, who called me right back. Joel's muscle and joint symptoms, in retrospect, were part of a paraneoplastic syndrome. "We were fooled", Dr. Fahler said. "The fall from the roof was a red herring. It was cancer pain all along."

Joel did get to ride his Harley-Davidson just a few times during the two short months of therapy he had before his cancer got the upper hand again.

24) TWO RED HERRINGS

Rodney Grussman is a mild-mannered, unassuming seventy-year-old man with diabetes, emphysema and valvular heart disease. I see him every three months to monitor his bloodwork and his symptoms. He sees his pulmonologist about twice a year and has a couple of nodules in his right lung Dr. Welch is following.

At his last three-month-visit everything seemed fine, except he was at the tail end of a cold, which seemed to have left him slightly short of breath. His exam was normal, his oxygen saturation hovered around his baseline, and we agreed that he would let me know if he didn't bounce back over the next week or so.

Almost two months later, Rodney came back to see me.

"Doctor, I am so winded. I have lost my stamina since I had that cold."

His exam was unchanged. I wondered if he could have had a silent heart attack or if something was going on with his lungs. His EKG was unchanged, but his chest x-ray suggested a couple of new, very small nodules in his left upper lobe.

I ordered an echocardiogram because of his leaky valve and referred him back to Dr. Welch for his opinion.

The echo showed no deterioration of Rodney's pump function; his ejection fraction was still 40%, just like three years ago. That is a little lower than the 55% considered normal. His valves looked about the same as two years ago.

I waited for Jerry Welch's report, but didn't hear anything for a while. Then I found out that he was trying to get insurance approval for a PET-scan because the new nodules in Rodney's left lung looked suspicious on a non-contrast CT scan. Due to his compromised kidney function, Rodney can't have intravenous contrast dye with his CT scans.

The PET-scan finally came back normal. Rodney came back to see me. His pulmonology report focused on the new lung nodules much more than Rodney's shortness of breath.

As I listened to Rodney's story again, it struck me: His heart was still decent, his lungs no worse than before, but what about the oxygen carrying capacity of his blood? A simple blood count showed he was quite anemic, and his stool test was positive for blood. He's getting his upper and lower endoscopy next week.

I hadn't considered all my ABC's from my emergency training - A for Airway, B for Bleeding and C for Circulation, although for more chronic conditions, perhaps it should be A for Anemia, B for Breathing and C for Circulation.

25) ANNIE LAUGHS WITH THE ANGELS

Nell and Gary Ruggles praised God for their firstborn after years of hoping and praying for a child. She was a small-boned and petite waif of a girl, with blonde fuzz on her head, a slightly reserved attitude and cautious, measured body movements. When Annie was happy, she blossomed, and could make the world smile with her musical laughter, but when she was unhappy, her weak little cry was heartbreaking.

The two of them gave Annie everything a little girl could want, and they showered her with love. They sang, read, played and did everything they could to offer her the best start in life she could have.

When Annie was a little over a year old, Nell became pregnant again, this time with twins. Gary couldn't have been more pleased. Coming from a large family himself, he pictured his children having the same experiences he cherished growing up with many siblings.

Around the time Sarah and Seth were born, Annie seemed to regress. She seemed less social, and she seemed to need more help than she had just the month before. She cried more, and seldom showed her exuberant side.

Their regular doctor suggested Annie might be jealous of the twins and just temporarily regressing, but Gary and Nell worried. A second opinion with a pediatrician in the city nearby concurred with their own doctor and suggested they give Annie more one-on-one time with each of them.

A few months later, Annie's deterioration was undeniable. Both doctors they had consulted now agreed there was something different about Annie, but didn't know what.

The doctors at City Pediatric Specialists were baffled. By now, the twins were catching up with Annie's development. Finally, a developmental specialist, who had studied under Dr. Andreas Rett, diagnosed Annie with Rett Syndrome just a few minutes into their consultation.

Just as they had been told, Annie became socially uninterested, almost always turned inward. She never smiled anymore. She developed unusual ways of holding her wrists and hands, chewed her fingers, stumbled and shuffled when she walked. She had already lost the ability to control her urine and bowels, and she stopped speaking. Her cry became even more heart shattering than it was in her infancy.

Today Annie is eight and a half. Her almost seven-year-old twin siblings help their parents take care of Annie. They keep the diaper supply stocked in the bathroom, bring toys within reach of Annie where she sits, put her mitts on when her hands get irritated by her gnawing, and take turns feeding her.

Annie seldom cries anymore. She shows little pleasure or displeasure. She shows almost no interest in Sarah and Seth, even when they clown around, trying to make her laugh.

But sometimes, in the middle of the night, Nell and Gary can hear her laughing in her room, a melodic laughter that sounds almost like bells chiming in the distance. As they listen hard, they sometimes even think they hear more than one note at the same time.

They say Annie laughs with the angels.

26) MEALS ON WHEELS

Arthur Bloch has slowly been losing weight over the past six months. His thyroid function and all his routine labs are normal. He has had a chest x-ray, and he had a colonoscopy and an upper endoscopy a couple of years ago. He says his appetite isn't what it used to be. He tells me he doesn't have any trouble swallowing.

His Parkinson's Disease is causing him to speak in a quiet, almost whispering voice, and his body movements and facial expressions are sparse. I have wondered if he might be depressed. He filled out a depression questionnaire a couple of months ago, and it was fairly unremarkable.

He and his wife, Zena, have had their share of health problems. Zena has become quite frail and has a mild dementia. Over the past few months, they have been set up with Meals on Wheels and homemaker services. Neither Arthur nor Zena drives anymore, and they are getting rides from the Senior Companion program. They usually come to each other's appointment, in fact they seem inseparable and very devoted to each other.

Today, Arthur happened to be in alone. Zena was at the hairdresser's. I reviewed his negative weight loss workup with him.

"I know why I am losing weight", he declared. I looked quizzically at him. He continued:

"It's the Meals on Wheels. Zena was always a wonderful cook and I ate like a king for fifty-two years, but with her dementia, she can't cook anymore. She feels bad about it, but we have no other choice except Meals on Wheels. I don't care for many of the meals, but I don't want to say anything. That would just hurt her feelings. So I say I'm not hungry."

"But you are hungry", I concluded.

"Yes." His eyes teared up.

"Can you get some desserts and instant breakfasts?"

"I suppose."

The mystery of Arthur's weight loss may be gone, but I am just as helpless with a diagnosis as I was without one.

27) HELPING PATIENTS ACCEPT THEIR "IMPERFECTIONS"

Brian was in a lot of pain, I could see it. But his lumbar MRI showed only modest changes. Two back surgeons said they couldn't help him. Physical therapy, chiropractic and osteopathy either didn't help or made him worse. Duloxetine helped only a little. After one day of a higher dose, he felt "loopy" and stopped it completely.

Then he found that marijuana helps a great deal. The only problem was that he started smoking a lot and began to act under the influence. His family didn't support him becoming a "pothead". His wife asked if there was anything other than duloxetine he could take.

A website that promised minimally invasive laser surgery several states away had caught Brian's attention. He asked me what I thought.

The same day I saw a woman who cries a lot.

Holly carries a diagnosis of bipolar disease. She is on one of the newer "atypical" antipsychotics. She functions pretty well, but told me she cries very easily: Movies, songs and good news can affect her. She doesn't feel sad, just the opposite, she cries more tears of happiness or empathy than of sadness or hopelessness.

She asked me if I knew of a medication for that.

In both cases I thought for a moment. Then I entered that mental space that gives me a sense of quiet authority and wisdom, as if I were speaking as a clergyman or a therapist.

"Brian", I said, "I don't think any medication will help you right now. You have your mind set on a surgical cure, and as long as you hold that vision, pills won't work for you."

He nodded in agreement.

"You gave up on the 60 mg dose after one single day of nonspecific side effects. You need to research the laser procedure."

He nodded again.

"But let me point this out to you: you've told me that marijuana makes you less stiff and makes your legs move better. That means you're not all rusted up. Marijuana does nothing to the bones, disks, muscles and ligaments in your body. The only thing it does is change how you experience things. If marijuana makes you limber, do you really need to have surgery, or can you change the pain experience through it and any other chemical or yoga, meditation, Reiki, prayer or whatever?"

His wife turned to him as if to ask him to answer me.

"The problem in your back can be overcome by changing how the nerves from your back and legs communicate with your brain. They are sending exaggerated signals that your back is completely broken when it really isn't. It has some glitches, but even smoking weed makes you able to use it with less pain, and the duloxetine starting dose did the same thing."

He looked straight at me and made a slight frown.

"But you're not ready to work on it that way. You will only be able to do that if you know for sure surgery can't make you "perfect". Go see the laser folks and talk to me again afterward."

I rose from my swivel stool and ended our visit. Brian and his wife seemed to exchange telepathic comments as they left the room.

"Holly", I said, "I could give you some Paxil and make you cry less, but you would very likely then also feel less joy and empathy. Is it worth risking losing a really good quality that you have?"

"No. I think of myself as a very empathic person. I would give my sweater to a cold homeless person, I'm like that."

"Right, you have bipolar disease, your mood may change quickly, but you are a very feeling person and maybe this world needs more people who can really feel things, be present in the moment."

"I like to be called a feeling person. I wouldn't want to not feel… I was just wondering if it is normal."

I held my hands out, palms up.

"It is normal. It can be beautiful."

She smiled and said "Thank you". Her eyes moistened as she got up from her chair.

I didn't offer any cures to these two, but I'm trying to help them see themselves as not some potentially flawless machines, but imperfect human beings, as we all are, who can still make the most of who they are and what they have.

28) A FIRE IN THE BELLY

Henry Halvorsen was in to see me the other day. 79 years old and usually brimming with optimism and vitality, he seemed subdued and frail. His weight loss and muscle weakness were obvious.

"Good to see you, it's been a long haul", I greeted him.

"Three surgeons, two CT scans, two hospital stays before they found out what was wrong with me, and then rehab and everything that happened there", he said, exasperated.

It had started when I saw him in the office at the end of February. He had been in three weeks earlier with a flare-up of his recurring back problem. That had cleared up, but Henry was having some bowel trouble, mostly constipation but then sometimes a day of loose stools. He thought it was his muscle relaxant that caused his bowels to act up, but his bowels didn't straighten out after he stopped his cyclobenzaprine.

He wasn't running a temperature, but his appetite was off. He was definitely a little tender deep in his right lower quadrant, but there was no involuntary muscle guarding when I let go of the pressure with my hands. I ordered bloodwork and a CT scan and told him that even though his pain and irregular bowels had been there for a whole week, he could have a subacute appendicitis.

His white blood cell count came back mildly elevated, and his sedimentation rate was elevated at 40 mm. The wait for the CT seemed long, but he was feeling better. Then, the day before his scan was scheduled, he woke up with worse pain and severe diarrhea, so he went to the emergency room. The ER physician, Jack Morton, told him right away he was suspicious of appendicitis.

His blood count was a little higher, and his sedimentation rate was 50. His abdomen was mildly tender, as it had been in my office. The CT scan showed no definite abnormalities, but the appendix was not visible.

The surgeon who saw him didn't feel there was quite enough reason to remove his appendix, and with intravenous fluids and bowel rest, Henry started feeling better. Another surgeon did a follow-up evaluation on the weekend and Henry was discharged home on the third day.

Two days later at one o'clock in the morning, he woke up with abdominal pain, followed by a very large, soft bowel movement. He had chills and felt nauseous. He called the ambulance and arrived at the emergency room actively vomiting.

Dr. Morton was on that night, too. He ordered the same bloodwork again and another CT scan. This time there were signs of a small bowel obstruction and free fluid in the abdomen. There were nonspecific inflammatory signs in the right lower quadrant but the appendix was not clearly identified.

The surgeon on duty that morning didn't hesitate. In short order Henry was on the operating table and had his ruptured appendix removed and two Jackson-Pratt drains placed. He received intravenous antibiotics and spent the next few days mostly sleeping with a Foley catheter draining his urine and a nasogastric tube draining his stomach.

At the rehab, where he was receiving intravenous antibiotics, he developed urinary retention shortly after his catheter was removed. The nurses were unable to reinsert a catheter due to his enlarged and inflamed prostate. Henry had to be transported back to the hospital where his urologist managed to get a Foley in. Then, back at the rehab, he developed diarrhea again and was diagnosed with Clostridium Difficile enteritis, resulting in more, but different, antibiotics.

As we went over everything that had happened to him, he sighed and said "I'm lucky to be alive".

I nodded and mused out loud. "It's such a common disease, but it can present in so many ways". I thought about the first CT scan and the first surgeon's decision not to perform an unnecessary operation.

I told him when I was a resident in Sweden, surgeons used to talk a lot about what percentage of innocent appendices you needed to operate on in order not to miss any guilty ones. Between 15 and 40 percent of emergency appendectomies have been reported to reveal a normal appendix, and yet 20 percent of appendicitis cases are initially misdiagnosed.

By the time I did my residency here, my hospital had just installed its first CT scanner, and the diagnosis of appendicitis was no longer a purely clinical one. In some centers, the diagnostic accuracy of CT scanning is said to be as high as 98 percent. But, when the tests are inconclusive or, worse, wrong, it is still a hard judgement call whether to operate or not.

Older patients tend to have less typical symptoms and are diagnosed later in the course of the disease than younger patients. While most cases of appendicitis fulminate within 48 hours, in 2 percent of cases the duration is more than two weeks.

"I'm just happy I pulled through", Henry said as he rose from his chair with obvious effort.

I shook his hand and answered, "I am, too, and we should all be humbled that the great trickster almost did it again."

29) CONTEXT, ALWAYS

Question: What do you do when presented with abnormal lab results?

Answer: Ask lots of questions.

The nursing home just sent over a urinalysis on a patient of Dr. Carlyle. I am covering his practice for a few days. The test showed that an 82 year old woman had 3+ white blood cells in her urine. "NKDA" was written in the margin, indicating she had no allergies.

I sighed internally and called the nursing home. The charge nurse seemed a little surprised at all my questions.

"What are the symptoms? What is the patient's kidney function? Is she on blood thinners or any other medications that might interact with an antibiotic?"

The presence of bacteria or white blood cells in the urine should not usually be treated if there are no symptoms. That's not always been our belief, but most doctors agree with this approach today.

Looking at a test result without knowing the story behind it, we cannot decide whether or how to act.

Last week we got a critically high potassium result on a patient with normal kidney function and no prescription medications in her profile. I did nothing about it, except order a repeat test that was normal. The obvious explanation was hemolysis; red blood cells contain more potassium than the serum that transports them and if the cells break during blood draw or handling of the vial, serum potassium will be falsely elevated.

A seizure patient of Dr. Carlyle had a high phenytoin level. I pestered the nurse to give me several past results and to track any previous dose changes. It turned out this patient had stable levels for a year and a half and suddenly had a low level last month. Dr. Carlyle raised the dose. In retrospect, the patient probably had missed a few doses, and would have been fine staying on the same dose. I dropped the prescribed dose back down and expect the patient to do fine.

A hypothyroid patient, Diane Green, was hospitalized with abdominal distention and constipation. She is nonverbal, and fearful of medical procedures. The hospitalist checked her thyroid function, as undertreated hypothyroidism can contribute to constipation. The test suggested Diane needed a higher dose, so she was discharged on a substantially increased dose of levothyroxine. As soon as I saw her again, I reversed the medication change; her TSH had been normal one week before her admission, and a severe illness or traumatic experience can affect thyroid values. I figured the hospitalist did not notice Diane's old TSH result in the hospital computer.

Context is crucial when deciding what to do with abnormal test results. But doctors are often pressed for time, and finding the story behind the results takes time. Even when all the data is in our electronic medical records, it takes time to see the patterns: The test results are usually in one place, the prescriptions in another, the office notes in a third, and the phone messages in a fourth. My own EMR can produce flowsheets with lab results, but each test is identified by the date it was ordered instead of the date it was performed, so correlating lab values with prescription dates becomes confusing, for example when following thyroid cases.

In times past, when solo practice physicians cared for their patients in the office, hospital and nursing home, they kept the threads of context and continuity together more easily. Today, with more providers sharing the care, and with other office staff also interacting with patients and their families, there is more room for errors, gaps and confusion. The tools we have right now are not always as effective as we would like, and they certainly can be cumbersome and slow to use. Reading each other's notes can take a while, as the EMR format is primarily built for coding and not for ease of following the clinical "story".

A few words doctor to doctor, doctor to nurse or doctor to patient can sometimes do what half an hour on the computer might not. Treatment without context is essentially just random reflex actions: Killing the innocent bacteria, lowering the falsely elevated potassium, treating the lab value and not the patient - none of it does anybody any good, and probably will cause harm to some unfortunate patients.

Our temptation to view test results as obvious facts in a predictable process instead of possibly misleading clues in a complex mystery reminds me of these words from a Sherlock Holmes novel:

"There is nothing more deceptive than an obvious fact."

Sir Arthur Conan Doyle

30) THE ART OF DIAGNOSIS

Arthur and Tom both had low testosterone and were prescribed testosterone replacement by their doctors.

In Arthur's case, it later turned out his low testosterone was just the tip of the iceberg; he was eventually diagnosed and treated by a Boston neurosurgeon for a pituitary tumor.

Tom's low testosterone, he found out too late to save his life, developed because his pituitary and almost every organ of his body was poisoned by iron due to hemochromatosis.

Early in my career I diagnosed Fran Dennison with hypertension and put her on lisinopril. She asked me to write her a 90-day prescription to save her money. As I always did, I ordered a creatinine and potassium level to be done the following week, and I asked her to come back in two weeks for a followup visit.

Three months later, I saw Fran again. She had never gone for the blood tests I had ordered. Her blood pressure was normal, 130/80, but she looked gravely ill. She was tired and nauseous, complained of leg cramps, had lost weight, and her skin had a peculiar yellow color. Unlike the last time she was in, her arterial pulses at the ankles seemed weak. I put my blood pressure cuff around her right calf and with my fingers on her posterior tibial artery I pumped the cuff up. When the sphygmomanometer reached 120, she winced, but I kept pumping, as the ankle pressure is usually significantly higher than the brachial pressure. In Fran's case, the ankle systolic pressure was 90 at best. As I listened with my stethoscope on her abdomen I heard a faint bruit over the aorta. I couldn't remember if I had listened the first time; there was no documentation of it in her chart.

Fran was in kidney failure from having a low blood pressure in the entire lower half of her body due to atherosclerotic narrowing of the aorta above the renal arteries. Before my blood pressure prescription, her leg muscles and kidneys had been adequately supplied with blood. If she had come in for her blood test, there would likely have been signs of early kidney stress, and she would have been spared months of suffering, but we did not track overdue lab results back then.

I stopped Fran's lisinopril, sent her for some STAT labwork and called the vascular surgery office at Cityside Hospital. They operated on her the next week, and her blood pressure normalized without treatment. I have been more diligent about listening for abdominal bruits and checking blood pressures at the ankles since then. I even got a Doppler soon after that in order to get the most accurate ankle blood pressure readings. I also never prescribe 90 days of lisinopril until the followup visit when I have seen the labwork.

Martin Brandt almost lost his leg one night in a small emergency room on the opposite side of Cityside Hospital. He was in the area visiting his sister when his left leg started hurting. The emergency room doctor ran many tests and gave Martin intravenous morphine, but even that barely controlled the pain. The surgeon on call finally made the diagnosis of an arterial embolus and almost six hours after his leg pain started, Martin had surgery at Downstate Hospital to remove the clot. He followed up with the vascular surgeons at Downstate and seemed to do well.

Four months later, when I saw him for a scheduled visit, I asked him if he was trying to lose weight. He had lost 20 lb. and admitted to feeling run down. He also had a possible hint of jaundice. His lab work confirmed that his bilirubin was elevated and after a CT scan showed dilated bile ducts and a possible pancreatic mass, I referred him to Cityside Gastroenterology for an ERCP. The stenting done during his procedure relieved the bile obstruction, but the biopsy showed pancreatic cancer. It isn't likely his prognosis would have been different if his tumor had been diagnosed along with his blood clot, but it is possible that it would have. Both arterial and venous blood clots can be paramalignant phenomena, but not every doctor thinks of that possibility.

There is an intense focus on the technical aspects of treatment in today's healthcare. The art of diagnosis is viewed as a quaint historical vestige in this era of advanced imaging and treatment protocols, and there seems to be less discussion about differential diagnosis than in years past.

We get caught up in the traps of self diagnosis or single dimension "diseases", like "low T" and irritable bladder. Even such common "diseases" as hypertension are really groups of diseases with similar symptoms but frighteningly different treatment and prognosis.

In today's fast paced medical office environment, how do we find the time and the mental space to step back and consider what might seem temptingly obvious with fresh and critical eyes - how do we manage to still practice and hone the Art of Diagnosis?

The chronicler of the vignette about Tom, the "low T" patient who died from his hemochromatosis, David A. Shaywitz, M.D., put it as well as anyone I have heard:

"The need to look beyond a patient's immediate clinical symptoms and to search intensively for deeper meaning has been and must always remain a defining quality of the medical profession."

31) LIFE AND DEATH

Elmer Ladd built the little pink house at the end of our road just in time for their wedding on New Year's Eve 1953. The pre-cut Aladdin home caught Elmer's eye when he first saw the catalog. Eileen picked the color and the two of them knew from the day they moved in that they would always live there, close to his work at the train station. Every day after the 12:05 had left, Elmer came home to eat lunch with Eileen. At precisely 12:50 he put his cap back on and left to greet the 1:05 southbound Express. Every afternoon when their daughters returned from school, Elmer was home again to spend a few minutes with them before returning to the station for the next train.

After Elmer retired from the railroad, he and Eileen spent all their time together at home, caring for the little pink house and the small garden. For the first few years he would still listen for the trains, but eventually he learned to ignore them. Ten years after his retirement the trains stopped running through our town and weeds grew quickly between the abandoned tracks.

One day a stray dog wandered into their yard, an off-white spaniel mix with brown spots scattered over her back. Eileen thought the dog looked like a large mushroom when she first noticed her through the kitchen window. They called her Mushroom, and she quickly filled the void they had both felt in their life.

With Mushroom two paces ahead, behind or to the side, Elmer did the rounds around town morning and afternoon. The sweet-tempered dog made friends along the way, and Elmer tipped his old uniform hat to passers-by and shopkeepers as they walked. He had found a purpose and a routine again, and he was thriving. He constantly talked with or about the dog, and called her his little girl.

Then the seizures began. The veterinarian was not able to control them with medication, and Eileen worried that Elmer wouldn't be able to get the dog back home again if she were to have a seizure on one of their walks. They stayed closer to home and Elmer's world got smaller again.

Mushroom, sweet and gentle as ever, seemed content to stay inside the house or in the yard. On warm summer afternoons she dozed under the white porch swing while Elmer and Eileen sipped lemonade in the shade. More and more often and without warning, the dog would suddenly start convulsing to the point of losing control of her bodily functions, and the helpless elderly couple would kneel beside her and quietly pray for each spell to end. After she came to, Mushroom would seem confused, docile and grateful to be near them. She would wag her tail quietly and put her muzzle in the nearest hand or lap and fall asleep.

Summer turned into fall, and then winter. As the seizures worsened and came more often, Eileen broached the subject of putting Mushroom out of her misery.

"But does she suffer?" Elmer asked.

"I don't know, but we mustn't be selfish if there is any chance that she is", Eileen replied.

"It's not for us to play God. He gives life and only He can take life away from any of his creatures." Elmer's voice almost failed him as he spoke back to his wife.

Weeks passed, and the seizures grew in intensity. On a cold January morning, Mushroom collapsed at the end of the driveway and seized more violently than she had ever done before.

"Elmer, you've got to take her to the vet. You can't let the poor dog suffer any longer." Eileen sobbed: "Can't you see it's time?"

Without saying a word, Elmer put on his hat and jacket and trudged through the freshly fallen snow to the dog who lay quivering down the hill from the house.

He lifted Mushroom and walked slowly back up the hill. As he approached the car, Eileen ran out to open the back door for him.

His face was dusky, his breathing wheezy, and he moaned quietly as he leaned into the vehicle with Mushroom, whose limbs hung flaccidly as he coaxed her into the crowded back seat of the small sedan. The dog snored and exhaled loudly.

Silently, Elmer put his arms around Eileen. She sobbed. Then he opened the driver's side door and sat down behind the wheel. Just as he turned the ignition, he took a deep breath as if he meant to say something. Then his head slowly nodded as his body fell, lifeless, over the steering wheel. The horn blared and the dog raised her head in the back seat.

Eileen reached in and tried to pull him away from the steering wheel. She managed to turn off the ignition and as she did, she knew her husband was gone. She acted quickly, but the ambulance crew pronounced the love of her life dead at the scene.

Mushroom came prancing down the street this afternoon, her spaniel tail and feathers waving in the warm breeze of what felt like the first day of spring. Ten paces behind came Eileen. The two of them make their rounds every day now the way Elmer and Mushroom used to. The new veterinarian in the next town seems to have found the right medication to control the dog's seizures, and life somehow goes on for Elmer's two girls.

32) NO BETTER

"No better" was the message I got last week about a sore toe, a stubborn cough and a case of C. Difficile diarrhea. All three messages were false alarms, misleading missives, inadequate information or whatever you want to call it.

After a few more questions, all three patients turned out to actually be doing much better than the messages suggested.

The octogenarian with the sore toe, which looked like gout to me, told me the exquisite pain she had experienced from the lightest touch was gone, the throbbing had subsided, and now there was just a strange itching deep inside her toe. The swelling was almost gone, and she didn't even flinch when I squeezed her toe. The two days of prednisone I had prescribed really seemed to have helped her. And, her uric acid level had come back elevated.

The man with a cough back in April had actually almost stopped coughing after a ten day course of antibiotics for his cough, sinus congestion and postnatal drip. But his symptoms had gradually started to come back. He hadn't refilled his prescription as I had told him he could, but decided to give it more time. Now he was almost back at square one. I told him to take another round of the antibiotic and expect to see him do well.

The poor woman with clostridium colitis had improved significantly, but wasn't quite back to normal. Her probiotic order had stopped when her metronidazole stopped and she turned out to have a fondness for tall glasses of cold milk. I had her restart her lactobacillus and give up the milk, and within two days her stools were formed.

In all three cases, one or two simple followup questions provided information that the prescribed treatments had actually worked fairly well. But in all three scenarios, either the patient or the person who took the message seemed to have an all-or-nothing mindset, almost like a "true or false" quiz, or "complains of/denies" click boxes in our electronic medical record.

This is a problem in healthcare today: Information is expected to be "discrete", "structured", or straightforward. But people and diseases are usually more nuanced than that. And without the nuances provided by a real patient narrative, we risk making deleterious treatment decisions.

Medical practice is not usually so algorithmic that simple yes or no answers can guide our treatment decisions. One person's yes is another person's no, depending on their expectations and a host of psychological factors.

Our job is to listen to the narrative and, only then, decide whether to follow the "yes" or the "no" arm of whatever algorithm we are trying to apply.

In this era of EMR click boxes and team based care, there is a real danger of seeking simple answers without listening to patients long enough to understand what they are trying to tell us.

We learned this in medical school and residency. EMR people and office staff didn't. We need to pause and think like doctors before we give knee-jerk responses to seemingly simple messages.

33) INHALER CURES GERD (?)

His heartburn was way out of control, even on maximum doses of pantoprazole and ranitidine. It burned all the way up behind his breastbone and he could feel the choking quality of the sticky acidity deep in his throat. He hurt and coughed after eating, so hard that he would vomit and lose his breath. What he vomited was mostly mucous. "It's like my esophagus is bubbling over", he described it.

If he missed a dose of either medication, his symptoms worsened within an hour. "So the medications must be doing something, but nowhere near enough", he told me.

A couple of years ago he had been turned down for an upper endoscopy because he also happened to have severe angina, and the gastroenterologist was concerned about his anesthesia risk.

"So I keep suffering", he sighed.

He had the head of his bed elevated, and he didn't eat spicy food or drink alcohol, but he did smoke. And he admitted to a "smokers cough", every morning with some light colored phlegm.

I listened. Something didn't fit. He talked too much about mucous.

"Would you be willing to try something?" I asked.

"Anything", he answered.

I listened to his lungs and recorded his Peak Expiratory Flow, 300, moderately below normal.

"You have COPD", I explained.

He raised his eyebrows.

"Chronic Bronchitis, one form of COPD, is defined as cough with phlegm more than two months out of the year. I'd like you to try an inhaler that reduces your phlegm production and improves your breathing."

I left the room and went to get an inhaler from the sample closet. I logged it in the EMR and showed him how the device works and said, "use this once a day and see me back in two weeks. It will help your 'smokers cough', but it may also do something for your heartburn. If not, we'll really have to put our thinking caps on".

Exactly two weeks later, after I knocked on the exam room door and entered, he rose from his chair with a big grin and stretched out his right hand.

"With that inhaler just once a day, my heartburn is completely gone."

I checked his Peak Flow, 420.

"And your breathing is better, too", I added.

"Yes, and my smokers cough."

I sat down.

"All these years, all the doctors I've seen, and you just listened for a few minutes and...gave me an inhaler. Was it not GERD?"

I told him what I thought.

"You've got bad acid reflux, no question, but you also, obviously, have chronic bronchitis. So we've helped your breathing and dried up your bronchial secretions, which were very significant and very bothersome. Some of them probably went down your esophagus, even if you weren't consciously swallowing them, and maybe caused some irritation."

I took a deep breath and continued:

"But the inhaler I gave you is called an anticholinergic. It doesn't just reduce secretions in your lungs. It is absorbed into the blood stream and can have anticholinergic effects elsewhere in the body. I once had a patient, an older man with an enlarged prostate, become unable to urinate and needing his bladder catheterized because the inhaler affected his bladder's ability to contract. We use anticholinergic pills to help the problems many women have with frequent urination. Medications with anticholinergic side effects, like amitriptyline, can also affect bowel contractions and cause constipation. But I've never seen that from an inhaler like the one I gave you."

He seemed almost spellbound, and I continued:

"I really didn't know if the inhaler would do much for your acid reflux, and I've never heard of it being used for that, but when I was young I had terrible heartburn from the hiatal hernia I didn't even know I had back then. This was before the kinds of medicines you take were invented, before omeprazole, the Swedish forerunner to pantoprazole, and before ranitidine. The only medicine that existed for stomach acid was - an anticholinergic. I still remember, it was called "ULCOBAN" [probably for 'ulcer banned'?], and I also still remember how dry my mouth used to be when I took it. But it worked.

So, it was just a gut feeling, no pun intended, that there might be a double effect from the anticholinergic inhaler, less mucous in your lungs and less acid in your stomach. And we lucked out."

I thought he'd never let go of my hand as he shook it on his way out

34) A BAD CASE OF CONGESTION

Friday was unusually hazy, hot and humid for our northern location. My last patient before lunch was a "double book". Nat Bruehl, an infrequent visitor to our clinic, had called about congestion and an irritated eye. Probably a case of conjunctivitis, everyone involved had concluded, and he was given an appointment within an already filled time slot for a "quick look".

"I brought my daughter to her high-risk obstetrician's appointment in Capital City Monday, and she made us drive with the blasted air conditioner on the whole way there and back. Ever since then my eyes seemed irritated", Nat explained. "I figured I got a cold in them. I took some cold pills that didn't do any good. Then, last night my right eye started to hurt like a son of a gun and now everything is a little blurry. I even had a hard time driving myself here."

I looked at his face. His right eye was red, and as I looked closer, I noticed his pupil was enlarged. As I directed my wall mounted light at his eye, the pupil remained dilated and I could see that the fluid behind his cornea was gray and cloudy, barely letting the light through.

I brought him out in the hallway to look at the vision chart.

"Start with your good eye", I asked him. Outside, lightning struck not far from the office. The earth shook and the fluorescent lights blinked.

He squinted and strained, and missed two letters on the 20/40 line. With his right eye, he couldn't even do 20/100.

"You've got a true emergency", I explained. "I think you've got a dangerous buildup of pressure in your eye because of an internal blockage - a case of acute glaucoma, and I want you to see an ophthalmologist today.

"But I couldn't drive to the city", Nat protested. "Not in this weather."

"I wouldn't want you to", I warned him. "You need to find somebody else to drive you." I also asked for his permission to bring in our head nurse and my own nurse, Autumn, to look at his eye. "I would like everyone here to see what you've got", I explained.

He agreed, and I showed his abnormal eye to our nurses.

I made a call to the nearest ophthalmologist, Mike Dube, but he was off and had signed out to Jeremy Sweet over at Cityside Hospital. After hearing my case description, Dr. Sweet's assistant gave Nate a 3 o'clock appointment.

"Now, don't try to drive all the way there yourself", I warned him. He agreed to find someone to drive him. I gave him directions and went back to my office to catch up on charts and grab a bite of my sandwich. Outside, the sky darkened as if night had already fallen.

The afternoon was a whirlwind. Other places may wind down on Friday afternoons, but not our clinic. Just before 5 o'clock there was a call from Dr. Sweet's assistant.

"You were right", she said. "He has a bad case of angle closure glaucoma and we are having a hard time getting his pressures down. It's 50 even in his good eye. That antihistamine-decongestant he took for three days is probably what did it. Good thing you caught this - we often see people like this bounce around a bit before getting diagnosed."

I thanked her and made sure to let the staff know about the callback. Flashes of lightning lit up the darkness outside, the thunder roared almost continuously, the floor vibrated and the rain beat hard against my office window as I finished my charts for the week.

35) ALL GOD'S CHILDREN

Joey Lafleur was in for his four-year well child check yesterday morning, and it was a profound moment in a day that was otherwise more or less a blur of acute visits and urgent phone calls.

Joey seemed different from other babies early on to his previous provider. His doctor was Barbara Brandon, my good friend and colleague, who ended up giving up her career as a doctor because of her own health. Her early office notes, referral letters and the various specialist reports read like a medical mystery novel.

Joey didn't reach his developmental milestones; his eyes didn't seem right and he had an unusual, broad grin, which he always flashed. By age two he was diagnosed with Williams Syndrome, a rare genetic disorder that affects one in 7,500 newborns.

Joey, in typical fashion for Williams Syndrome children, is extremely gregarious, even with strangers. He is a favorite with the nurses. He isn't potty trained, cannot make three word sentences, and cannot make age-appropriate drawings.

His parents elected to give him the 4-6 year-old shots yesterday, and he protested loudly. Immediately afterward, he wanted to kiss the nurses.

Yesterday afternoon I saw Marguerite Brown, an eighty-three year old woman with stubborn blood pressure and skin problems. Two months ago she had told me that her daughter, Molly DeLorme, had been diagnosed with inoperable cancer. I have been Marguerite's doctor for ten or fifteen years, and never realized that her daughter was the woman who wallpapered our house a couple of years ago; after all these years practicing in this community I am still finding out that people I have known for years are related to each other.

Last week I had seen Molly's obituary in the paper. The same issue of our local paper had a little "In Memoriam" piece about a six-year-old patient of mine, who drowned several years ago. His parents are still struggling with their loss.

Marguerite Brown was somber, naturally, as I entered the exam room.

"Why did Molly have to die, why couldn't it have been me?" she asked, rhetorically.

Tonight I answered two separate telephone calls from my children. Both of them are dealing with the consequences of choices they have made in the past. I have wished for a long time that I could have spared them what they are going through right now, but I am wise enough to know that most of us have to learn things for ourselves, and cannot learn from the mistakes of our parents.

I can imagine the heartache of Joey Lafleur's parents as they imagine what his life will be like, growing up with Williams Syndrome. I can imagine their grief as they think about all the things he will never do.

We must all remember that our children are only loaned to us. We have a natural desire to see them grow up to be healthy and happy, and more often than not I think we hope they will be a lot like us. Our task and privilege as their parents is to see them for who they are, and help them reach their potential.

A youngster with Down's or Williams Syndrome can be more capable of receiving and returning the love of their parents than a child without genetic challenges, and a healthy child can be killed in a freak accident in the matter of seconds. The wisest parents cannot protect their children from making their own mistakes, and even the elderly often have to grieve the loss of a child.

36) ENDOCARDITIS OR NOT? A SATURDAY TRIAGE DECISION

Saturday clinic. No lab. Just me and a medical assistant.

A fifty year old woman comes in with a fever a couple of days after a dental cleaning. Her gums are sore and she has some bodyaches. I've never seen her before. She used to see Dr. Wilford Brown and transferred to Dr. Kim.

The inflammation in her mouth is mild. She has a Grade 1 holosystolic murmur. Nobody has documented that before, but a Grade 1 is usually insignificant and barely worth documenting.

The only other thing I notice on her exam is that she has two thin brown lines under one of her fingernails. Like splinter hemorrhages. But there are only two.

"I banged that finger by accident a month ago, I'm pretty sure those lines have been there since way before my dental cleaning", she said.

"Hmm, how bad are your bodyaches?"

"I'm not a complainer, I guess you could call them pretty bad."

Time to make a decision. A judgement call: Hospital for blood cultures, possibly IV antibiotics, or blame the whole thing on a sore mouth and a virus and an incidental fingertip injury. One explanation or three?

Logic seemed to dictate one explanation for three clinical signs: mouth, fever, fingernail. But then there are bodyaches, bad bodyaches.

I made my decision, explained it carefully, and she concurred.

"So, stop in first thing Monday morning for some bloodwork, pick up the prescription I'm sending to the pharmacy, and call us if you don't hear back from me by 10 am", I said.

I slept well for two nights and did my Sunday farm chores without thinking much about it.

Monday, 9 am:

Lowish white blood cell count, close to 50% each of lymphocytes and neutrophils.

"I got your bloodwork. How are you feeling?"

"Fine, my mouth feels great and the fever is gone."

"The blood count looks very typical for a virus."

Minor mouth infection, viral illness and a banged fingertip. Bingo.

37) A PEARL FROM MEDICAL SCHOOL

In Sweden, back when I trained, three blood tests were the "routine labs" done at most doctor visits: Hemoglobin, White Bloood Cell Count and Erythrocyte Sedimentation Rate. I'm trying to remember, but I don't think everyone waited an hour to see the doctor, so they must have used a modified rapid sedimentation rate.

The "Sed Rate", or "sänkan" as we call it, was invented by Robin Fåhraeus, a relative of one of my High School teachers. Fåhraeus described the phenomenon in his doctoral dissertation in 1921 and was professor of anatomy and pathology at Uppsala University around the time I was born. He was nominated for the Nobel prize several times but was never awarded it. He collaborated with another Swede, Alf Westergren, on perfecting the technology. Blood in a vertical tube will separate into liquid on top and clumped together red blood cells on the bottom. The height of the fluid pillar after one hour is the "sedimentation rate".

Anyway, in Sweden we were often faced with what to do when the sedimentation rate was abnormally high. In addition to the usual causes like infection, autoimmune disorders and multiple myeloma, it was drilled into my head to look for kidney cancer.

I've never heard any of my American colleagues talk about that, although there are several articles about the connection if you Google it.

A few weeks ago I saw a man who wasn't feeling well. I ordered some lab tests, including a sed rate. It came back at 100 mm, five times the normal limit. I ordered a CT of his abdomen to look for kidney cancer. Before he ever got the test, he ended up in the emergency room with pneumonia. That could have explained the abnormal lab result. Because of the severity of his pneumonia, the hospital did a chest CT on him, so when he got the call about his appointment for the abdominal CT I had ordered, he told them he didn't need it because he already had one. He thought one CT covered everything.

At his followup appointment, he was back to feeling nonspecifically unwell and his sed rate was now 118. I asked him to please reschedule his abdominal CT.

Today I got the result, a "Code Yellow, Unexpected Finding" fax in my office chair.

He has a one inch tumor in his right kidney, highly suspicious for cancer.

38) A REALLY BAD BRUISE

Theodore Black woke up two weeks ago with a massive bruise from the left side of his chest to his lower abdomen. He ended up admitted to the intensive care unit and wasn't discharged from the hospital until today.

"Cough and rash", was his chief complaint in my clinic schedule that morning. I had an emergency room report from Lakeside Hospital, near where he had spent a week at a conference. Two days before I saw him, he had gone to Lakeside's ER with a nasty cough and pain across his lower chest and upper abdomen, radiating all the way around his mid-back like a vice. They got a normal chest X-ray, and a normal complete blood count and chemistry profile, so they sent him out with prescriptions for pain pills and some cough medicine.

"I've still got this really bad cough, and the pain hasn't let up", he started, "and when I woke up this morning, I had this rash..."

He lifted his shirt and exposed a massive bruise running along the left side of his body from the level of his nipple to his hip.

My mind raced into action as I listened to his heart and lungs, palpated his lymph nodes, examined his abdomen by inspection, auscultation, palpation and percussion. His breath sounds were slightly diminished at the base of his left lung, the bruised area was dense and extremely tender. His abdomen wasn't very tender, except under the bruise, but he had some flank dullness on the right. He hurt too much on the left side to let me percuss him there, and he was unable to roll over on his left side to allow me to check if the right-sided dullness to percussion shifted with a change in position.

His blood pressure was a little lower than usual, but his pulse was low - which was to be expected with the beta blocker he takes for his blood pressure.

I couldn't remember the eponym for what he had, but I knew he had massive internal bleeding somewhere. In the back of my mind I thought I remembered retroperitoneal bleeding from coagulopathy or cancer, necrotizing pancreatitis or possibly intraabdominal bleeding.

I ordered a fingerstick prothrombin time, which came back normal at 1.0 and a CBC and a chemistry profile which I knew would be ready in just a few minutes with our new chemistry analyzer. I told him I'd be back as soon as the labs were done.

Back in the office I googled "flank ecchymoses" and saw the eponym I had forgotten, Grey Turner's Sign. Everything I remembered or just instinctively knew about it matched the monograph I found.

His CBC came back first, and his hematocrit had dropped from 40 at Lakeside to 27 - definitely a massive bleeding. I went back in his room and told him that I not only wanted him to go to the hospital but that I didn't want him going all the way there in a private car, but in the ambulance. Just as Autumn was calling the emergency dispatch number, Ted's chemistries came back, with the lowest sodium level I have ever seen, 116 mg/deciliter. It had been 140 two days earlier.

I have seldom seen symptomatic hyponatremia, and the correlation between sodium levels in the brain and in peripheral blood isn't very predictable, but the literature suggests that people with sodium levels as low as Ted's are likely to be obtunded or having seizures. He seemed quite normal in that regard. Still, it made me feel good about my decision to recommend that he should go to the hospital via ambulance.

Ted had a chest CT angiogram, showing a modest amount of blood in his left chest cavity, but there was no bleeding or any other abnormality in his abdomen or pelvis on those scans. His pancreas and kidneys looked just fine. They slowly corrected his sodium deficiency and watched him carefully, but he didn't lose any more blood and he had no seizures or any other neurological symptoms. In the end, after his long and likely very expensive hospital stay, he was discharged for the second time on pain pills and strong cough medicine.

The final diagnosis was "Hyponatremia secondary to volume loss from left hemothorax and extensive ecchymoses from severe cough".

I had expected to hear bad news any day from the hospital, but my first and possibly only sighting of Grey Turner's Sign turned out to be very benign. My colleagues were aware of my initial observations and this afternoon I walked around and told them how things had turned out.

"I'm sure someone will write that case up and publish it", Dr. Brown said, probably referring to one of the major medical journals. "Definitely", I answered. I never did get around to telling Dr. Brown that I am writing this blog.

So, if The New England Journal of Medicine runs a piece on hyponatremia due to severe internal hemorrhage from coughing, you read it here first.

39) A DOCTOR'S PARTING WORDS

We are settling in back home tonight after a two-week trip to New York City and one of the Mid Atlantic states. We stayed at one hotel for twelve nights and it started to feel like a home away from home. This was the first trip for our puppy, a black German Shepherd, who actually turned one year old while we were away. This dog makes friends everywhere we go.

I am not as gregarious as our puppy, but at this particular hotel I made friends (sometimes because of the dog) with all the desk clerks and the newly hired maintenance man and his helper. I also had a quiet understanding with the woman who ran the complimentary breakfast buffet. I never took the dog there, but he contributed to my multiple trips to the free buffet every morning. This dog doesn't eat dog food; we feed him human grade food, so I made a few trips every morning to the breakfast buffet to load up on eggs and bacon for the dog and me, as well as pastries and yogurt for my wife.

Every morning the breakfast buffet supervisor seemed to look me over as I heaped a generous amount of eggs and bacon on my plate and disappeared to our room, only to appear minutes later for another big helping. She always smiled at me and said with an East-European accent: "Have a nice breakfast". Whenever I ran into her somewhere else in the hotel, she smiled as if she knew my little secret and always said something nice.

Early this morning, after three trips downstairs to pack the car, as we passed through the lobby on our way out for the last time, it seemed as if they were all there. The night desk clerk, just coming off duty, the daytime desk clerk, the maintenance man, even the breakfast lady showed up, seemingly to say good-bye to the puppy. The breakfast lady was the last one to do so, and she spoke to Moses in Russian.

I said, in Russian, mustering all I could remember from thirty years ago: "I understand a little Russian".

She beamed, exclaimed "Ochen chorosho (very good)!" and went into something long and complicated, of which I understood nothing. I reverted to English and told her why I came to learn some Russian at all when I did my military service back in Sweden.

She smiled and said softly "I am doctor in Russia, here - " and she shrugged, "housekeeping".

I wanted to say something more profound and supportive, but the puppy was starting to get impatient, we were already an hour behind schedule and we had a very long drive ahead of us. All I could do was mumble something about reading somewhere that there are many foreign-trained doctors who are having trouble getting their license here. Then I drove back home to my life as a doctor in America while she went back to check on the breakfast buffet.

40) MAGNESIUM DEFICIENCY - AN UNRECOGNIZED PANDEMIC LINKED TO TODAY'S CHRONIC DISEASE EPIDEMICS

A patient who hadn't felt good for many years came in the other day and told me an osteopathic physician she had gone to for OMT, manipulative treatment, had suggested she take two capsules of a basic 400 mg magnesium supplement every day and it had been life changing for her.

She handed me a xeroxed little essay the osteopath had written about the many functions of magnesium in the human body and the symptoms of deficiency.

All her vague gastrointestinal symptoms were gone, her skin had cleared, her energy level had improved and she felt more clearheaded.

"What was your level?" I asked.

"He didn't check it" was her answer.

I didn't know what to think, I mean it's probably harmless to take, but without knowing the level...

I started looking into this and the more I read, the more intrigued I became.

I found several articles from the last century (the 1990's) all the way up to last week (news that excess vitamin D can lead to osteoporosis, apparently through lowering bone magnesium levels), all saying mostly the same things:

Even though magnesium is abundant on this planet, many people (for example 80% of postmenopausal women with osteoporosis) have low intracellular magnesium. Almost half the US population consume less than the recommended daily amount of magnesium.

Serum levels of magnesium tell us nothing about total body magnesium, because we are programmed to pull magnesium from our tissues to keep blood levels in range. Only 1% of our body's normal 25 grams of magnesium is found outside our cells, and about 90% is found in bone and muscle cells.

Magnesium is essential for the function of 300 enzymes, mitochondrial ATP production and activation (cellular energy), synthesis of DNA, RNA and protein and regulation of ionic gradients (keeping sodium and potassium levels normal).

Magnesium deficiency is linked to inflammation (as measured by C-Reactive Protein, CRP), atherosclerosis, vasospasm, insulin resistance and metabolic syndrome as well as isolated hypertension.

Magnesium deficiency has been linked to sudden cardiac death.

The magnesium content of ur modern diet is decreasing, because of more and more processing of food as well as modern farming practices and soil depletion; we are also consuming things like phosphorus (in soft drinks) that lower body magnesium levels.

According to the NIH:

"Early signs of magnesium deficiency include loss of appetite, nausea, vomiting, fatigue, and weakness. As magnesium deficiency worsens, numbness, tingling, muscle contractions and cramps, seizures, personality changes, abnormal heart rhythms, and coronary spasms can occur. Severe magnesium deficiency can result in hypocalcemia or hypokalemia (low serum calcium or potassium levels, respectively) because mineral homeostasis is disrupted."

Not only can low magnesium contribute to the development of diabetes, but there are indications that magnesium supplementation may improve blood sugar control in diabetics. Magnesium supplementation has been shown to improve lipid profiles. Other not yet certain possible benefits of magnesium supplementation are migraine prevention and asthma control.

People at risk for magnesium deficiency, besides diabetics, include the elderly, patients taking diuretics or Proton Pump Inhibitors, those with inflammatory bowel disease or chronic diarrhea from other conditions, patients who have had small bowel surgery, people with gluten sensitivity and patients with alcohol or soft drink dependence. Perhaps surprisingly, people who exercise vigorously can also become magnesium deficient.

Foods that supply good amounts of magnesium include almonds (check), spinach (check), black and kidney beans (check) and avocado (check), and also some things that aren't on my meal plan: Peanuts, soy milk, shredded wheat, bread (presumably whole grain) and yogurt.

So, this is from someone who usually doesn't think much of vitamins and supplements: Because I've been taking PPIs for my hiatal hernia since they first came out and because my blood pressure is higher than I'd like in spite of being pretty ideal weight - I picked up a bottle of magnesium capsules the other day.

And the more I read, the more I worry about the decreasing nutrient value of much of our mass produced foods. The BMJ points out:

"The loss of magnesium during food refining/processing is significant: white flour (−82%), polished rice (−83%), starch (−97%) and white sugar (−99%). Since 1968 the magnesium content in wheat has dropped almost 20%, which may be due to acidic soil, yield dilution and unbalanced crop fertilisation (high levels of nitrogen, phosphorus and potassium, the latter of which antagonises the absorption of magnesium in plants)."

41) A FAILED TRANSITION OF CARE

Alvion Barr had a four month delay in his diagnosis.

He is technically a patient of my colleague, Dr. Laura McDonald. But he had drifted between two of our regular doctors and a locum tenens physician we hired to work during March, when both Laura and Dr. Wilford Brown were on vacation.

I saw him late Thursday afternoon for a rash, but he also asked what he could do about his heartburn.

"Tell me more about your heartburn", I said.

What followed was a near classic description of angina pectoris. He had been getting progressively more short of breath with exertion since Christmas, and if he didn't slow down when he started to get winded, he would get a dull pain in the middle of his chest that gradually spread to his jaw.

Alvion's problem list read like a Who's Who of vascular diseases and interventions: Coronary artery disease with a prior bypass operation and two stents a couple of years later, surgical repair of an abdominal aortic aneurysm, bilateral carotid bruits and mild intermittent claudication. He is also a diabetic and he quit smoking only two years ago.

"I have an appointment with the lung doctor next week to go over all the testing he just put me through", Alvion said.

I checked his peak flow. It was 550, same as mine.

"When was your last stress test", I asked him.

It became evident that he wasn't the best historian.

"Just a month or two ago, and it was okay."

"Do you remember who ordered it?"

"Dr. McDonald, I think."

Our EMR had no stress test result, not even an order for a stress test.

Health InfoNet, the statewide Internet repository of test results and hospital records, did have a nuclear stress test report from March 21 of this year, done at Cityside hospital.

My eyes scanned their way down the report and as I read the conclusion, I could feel the hair on the back of my neck rising:

"Large, reversible anterolateral defect...."

"March 21", I said out loud as I scanned the Health InfoNet site. "Here it is: Hospital discharge, March 21". We did have that document in our own record also. I continued reading out loud: "Final diagnosis: Non-Cardiac chest pain."

Alvion's troponins had been negative and the EKG portion of his stress test had been normal. There was no report from the nuclear images, but there was a comment, indicating that the images were of poor technical quality and that a final report would not be forthcoming for that reason.

He was prescribed pantoprazole for acid reflux, and here he was in my office after five o'clock on a Thursday afternoon four months later with classic, frequent although not crescendo angina and a highly abnormal stress test.

He had had a hospital followup with the locum tenens doctor, a Transition of Care visit as we now call them. We have created a template to meet the Medicare criteria for the new transition of care codes 99495 and 99496. One of the items is "Pending results at discharge:". In Alvion's case the word after the colon was "None".

I started Alvion on isosorbide mononitrate, a long acting nitroglycerin. He was already on a beta blocker, a statin and a blood thinner. I made sure he had more sublingual nitroglycerin and told him not to push himself and to call 911 if he had chest pain that didn't go away after two nitroglycerins.

The next morning I called the cardiology office and happened to get to talk to the doctor who had read the nuclear images after the patient had already left the hospital. He took no responsibility for the confusion. All he had to say was "I thought the hospitalist would contact the patient in a case like this".

"If he was on duty when the report came in", I thought, adding to myself "and if he read through the whole thing, since you had already told him it was uninterpretable".

42) NOAH'S JOURNEY

John and Elizabeth Tuttle had only one son. Noah was born with pneumonia and he didn't look like other babies. His nose was thin and his ears were pointed. He was very small and he didn't cry the way other babies do.

Noah never learned to speak in full sentences and he never grew up to find his own way in the world. He stays at home with his mother and father and spends most of his time playing quietly with his toy animal collection, his sticker books and his View Master 3-D pictures. He always seems happy and always has hugs and kisses for his parents.

Noah is now fifty years old.

A few years ago he developed pancreatitis and had to stay in the hospital for almost two weeks. He cried for his parents, who, both in their eighties, were too exhausted to stay with him in the hospital all the time.

I visited Noah on the surgical ward during that time, and I can still vividly see the image of the small, elderly-looking man with a plush zebra in bed with him, his hands without wrinkles or calluses, his face without beard growth and his eyes so deep and sad.

"You my doctor!" He smiled when he recognized me.

"How are you feeling, Noah?" I asked.

"Noah's sick" was all he said.

"You'll be okay soon; you'll be home soon", I promised.

John Tuttle is a soft-spoken man with a thick Yankee accent, who never wastes his words. He hates to take pills, and he is on several. He should be on more because his blood pressure is still too high. He blames it on stress and I agree that his plate is full. Once, about a year ago, he spoke to me of his biggest fear:

"I worry about Elizabeth's heart and I worry about Noah. What will happen to him after we're gone? I hate to think of him in an institution. He's always been with us."

A few months ago Noah suddenly gained weight. His legs swelled and he became short of breath. His chest x-ray showed only a mild enlargement of his heart, but his echocardiogram showed a severe weakness of his heart muscle and a critical aortic stenosis. The main valve of his heart was closing and choking his entire circulation.

After a few days in the hospital he was breathing comfortably again, but he was homesick and cried when his parents weren't there.

There had been no warning. There was no heart murmur. Noah had always lived a very sedentary life. His aortic valve had calcified without causing the usual symptoms until he became short of breath just playing in his room.

The chief of cardiology, Dr. Thomas Wentworth, said that an aortic valve replacement could be done, but because Noah's heart was so weak there was little hope that it would recover. It was not likely his symptoms would go away by just replacing the valve.

I met with John and Elizabeth shortly thereafter. They had made up their minds not to put Noah through open-heart surgery with such an uncertain outcome. They wanted us to manage Noah's heart failure with medications.

Noah is out of the hospital. He takes several new medications and is breathing comfortably. Noah talks about not liking the hospital. He stays at home with his mother and father and spends most of his time playing quietly with his toy animal collection, his sticker books and his View Master 3-D pictures. He always seems happy and still has hugs and kisses for his parents.

John and Elizabeth wonder quietly whose journey will end first.

43) TOO MANY CHEST PAINS

There are at least 50 words in the Eskimo languages for snow, 25 in mainstream Swedish, and supposedly 180 or so in the Sami language of the nomadic inhabitants of the northernmost parts of Norway, Sweden and Finland.

But there are even more words than that for "chest pain" among my patients, many of whom do not consistently or fully comprehend the English phrase "If you have chest pain, call 911 or go to the nearest emergency room".

This Saturday I had three serious cases of chest pain, but of course they all used different words, like "empty feeling", "tightness" and "pressure".

"The medical term is PAIN", I patiently explained to all three. They all had normal EKGs. "Thirty years ago that would have been more reassuring than it is today", I told each one of them. "But today we have blood tests that can show heart muscle damage that doesn't ever show up on an EKG. So today's standard of care is that you get to the emergency room where they can do these blood tests."

One patient got pain free after a "GI cocktail", which numbed his irritated esophagus, so I agreed to leave it at that, with a caution that new pains might require urgent reevaluation. Another agreed to go to he ER, declined the ambulance and seemed to understand my concern that his wife could find herself transporting a medical emergency patient singlehandedly on a winding road with sketchy cell phone reception. His wife also understood. The third patient accepted the ambulance, and left the building accompanied by the attendants, only to part company with them in the parking lot.

My compliance officer, after I told her we've got to figure out how to discourage Walk-in chest pains with our Saturday skeleton crew, asked about legal risk when the two most recent cases declined the ambulance. I wasn't worried; the first one I counseled thoroughly, and the second one left the building in the company of EMS. Once EMS takes over, my responsibility ends, that's well established, no matter what qualifications the doctor in the field has.

We have posters, pamphlets, mailings and all kinds of communications that encourage coming to see us for nonemergent medical problems like coughs, sprains, earaches, rashes and the like but to quickly get ER care for chest pain, severe shortness of breath and other dramatic symptoms.

Every month at our Quality Assurance meeting we look at how many ER visits in our patient population could likely have been handled in the office instead. I don't have statistics on how many people delay care for a serious cardiopulmonary condition by insisting to be seen by us first, but it sure happens.

We definitely need to do more training with front desk staff about this, but I know many patients will not admit to the receptionist that what they have is chest pain; they will try some of the other words instead.

So before Saturday, I think I'll have to come up with some new, catchier posters about the fact that they all mean the same thing: PAIN.

And that in turn means: NOT HERE.

44) SHADOW SYNDROMES

A fellow country doctor and blogger wrote a piece the other day about drug companies pushing medications for near-diseases like prediabetes and heartburn. I agreed with his sentiments and went on to think a lot about this. There is a tendency among drug companies and even some doctors (perhaps looking for business?) to medicalize the human experience. We all have heartburn sometimes, but is it a disease or pre-disease, or did we simply eat too much of the wrong kind of food?

I have mentioned before on my blog that Thomas Moore, the scholar and philosopher about matters of the soul, has said that book titles on your shelf can be inspiring even if you haven't read the book.

A couple of years ago, at a Harvard psychiatry or psychopharmacology course, the booksellers in the lobby had a book that caught my imagination and has been an inspiration to me from that moment, even though I didn't start to read it until today. It is by John Ratley, MD (co-author of "Driven to Distraction") and Catherine Johnson, PhD (author of "When to Say Goodbye To Your Therapist"). The title says it all: "Shadow Syndromes" (The Mild Forms of Major Mental Disorders That Sabotage Us).

People with near-diseases can benefit from comparisons with the full-blown thing only if the analogy provides them with a deeper understanding of their situation and a course of action to change their trajectory away from the disease they are heading towards. This applies to labels in general. Labels are good if they help you understand what's going on, and bad if they lock you into some sort of fixed category where you either don't believe you can get out or, perhaps worse, start to feel comfortable and liberated from your own responsibility for your life and health.

Somehow in the last generation of doctors, we seem to have lost our ability, or perhaps our perceived right, to give patients advice about their health; only if we diagnose them with a disease, or pre-disease, do we have something to tell them. We need to re-claim our position as health coaches, and fight for our right to tell people who are not yet diagnosable with an illness how to stay away from disease, instead of trying to make almost or completely healthy people carry a disease label, just so we can talk to them about how to stay out of trouble in the future.

45) THREE DUTCHMEN WALKED INTO AN EYE CLINIC, AND THE REST IS HISTORY

As a severe myopic, it is no wonder I have always had a certain interest in ophthalmology. And just the other day I had reason to ponder the peculiar Dutch dominance in the history of optics and ophthalmology.

When I was a nearsighted young school boy in Sweden, my mother brought me on the bus into town every fall to see the eye doctor. He must have been in his eighties, a tall man with a bow tie and a long white lab coat. His office was adjacent to his apartment in a white stucco building from the early 1900's. It was a dimly lit space with dark, angular furniture. The doctor said very little as he made me read the letters on the Snellen eye chart while placing varying lenses in front of each of my eyes in an antique looking device, and while he peered into my eyes while holding a thick magnifying lens that focused a piercing light into my tearing eyes one by one. I could smell his skin and his hair as he leaned into me.

After each of my annual exams, he always sighed and wrote out a stronger eyeglass prescription with a old black fountain pen. He carefully blotted the prescription paper and always said to my mother "don't let him read too much in bed".

As my glasses got stronger, I became aware that if I looked at road signs or traffic lights out of the corner of my eye, the colors didn't line up. The red outer circle of the Swedish no-parking signs would overlap one end of the inner blue circle and there would be a space between the two colors on the opposite side. In the same way, the red, yellow and green traffic lights wouldn't be straight on top of each other, but at an angle. I learned in school that red light passes straighter than blue or green light through a prism, like the outer edges of my old-fashioned glass lenses.

As I approached my teens, working with an old viewfinder camera and black and white darkroom equipment, I understood why it was harder to read in dim light: a dilated pupil, just like a wide aperture, creates a shallower depth of field than a smaller one, and the ultimate small aperture, a pinhole, can replace the lens in a simple camera or even your high powered eyeglasses in a pinch.

In medical school I learned to do a neurologic exam, and the bedside test for visual fields - Donders' confrontation, as we called it. I figured Donders was a Dutch name, but never gave it much thought.

The other night, wondering why my EMR incorrectly defines visual acuity by "Snelling" rather than Snellen, it struck me that Snellen was probably a Dutch name, just like Donders. A few minutes with my iPad and Dr. Google made me rediscover how much I enjoy medical history.

It turns out Donders built an eye clinic and hired Snellen to run it. They invited their friend Einthoven, who would later invent the EKG, to help in their research. Einthoven studied chromostereopsis, the phenomenon whereby red objects seem closer than blue objects. Donders, Snellen and their wives were the subjects, and Einthoven's paper became his doctoral thesis. It seems that chromostereopsis has something to do with the fact that red light travels straighter and that our eyeballs are angled inward when we look at objects up close, which makes blue objects seem ever so slightly blurry.

So, anyway, my little exploration reaffirmed that if I ever cut back my clinic hours, I'll read more about the history of medicine.

46) APPENDAGITIS, NOT A TYPO

A couple of years ago I saw a young man with pain in his lower right abdomen. I sent him for an urgent CT scan with a "wet read" to check for appendicitis.

It was afternoon and things were crazy at the office. I forgot all about the pending CT report. I have learned this about myself: I am efficient because I have the ability to hyperfocus, but that has made me dependent on my support staff to see the big picture of my schedule or pending, unfinished tasks.

The next morning there was a fax from Cityside with a lengthy explanation saying he had an epiploic appendagitis, and it went on to explain that this is a harmless and self limited condition.

I did some reading. These appendages are little fat bumps that run along the outside of the colon. They can undergo torsion, or twisting, and become acutely inflamed. This condition is found in up to 7% of patients suspected of having appendicitis and 1% of patients with suspected diverticulitis.

I had never heard of appendagitis, and I wondered how certain the distinction was between this harmless and the other potentially lethal -itis was.

Checking with the patient, he was in more pain and more nauseous than the day before.

I suggested going to the ER just to make sure. I just didn't feel comfortable trusting a CT and a diagnosis I had never heard of. I imagine this is a result of training before CT scans were in use and then not rubbing elbows enough with major surgery to be aware of the finer distinctions of the differential diagnosis in acute abdomens already too sick for the primary care office.

The ER report from Cityside was gracious in its description of why my young patient was there. He got an anti inflammatory medication and some pain pills and went home reassured. He was still uncomfortable when we called him a day later, but feeling better.

The other day I saw a young woman who had been to Mountainview Hospital for left lower quadrant abdominal pain.

She had a history of diverticulosis, and at her young age had already had a CT proven episode of acute diverticulitis a few years earlier. This time, the CT showed a sigmoid epiploic appendagitis with no evidence of diverticulitis. The ER doctor prescribed antibiotics that would have been appropriate if she had diverticulitis.

I saw her two days after the emergency room visit. She was feeling a bit better. Her exam was benign and I explained to her that she didn't really need the antibiotic. But I also told her it was a rare condition that I had not heard of in my first 35 years of practice. I told her the Mountainview ER doc probably hadn't seen a case before either, or didn't trust the CT.

My patient was happy to stop her antibiotics and happy that her diverticular disease was not the cause of her symptoms.

You're never too old to learn.

47) A MOVING TARGET

He was a new patient. His medical records described him as severely hearing impaired and suffering from a rare movement disorder. He arrived with a caseworker for his 11:30 first appointment and I was running late.

"Why is a new patient or a minor surgery procedure ever scheduled at the end of the morning instead of at the beginning", I asked Autumn, rhetorically.

The man seemed to be bouncing around in the small exam room. His head bobbed randomly and his body moved like waves in a wading pool full of three-year olds.

I introduced myself. His caseworker, clipboard in her left hand, shook my right hand. The man floated toward me, cocked his head suddenly and hollered while pointing to his right ear:

"I can't hear!"

"For how long?" I asked.

He didn't seem to hear me.

"At least a few years from what I know", his caseworker answered, drowned out by the man's repetition, "I can't hear, I can't hear!"

He seemed irritable, frustrated, and there was an air of desperation in the room. The caseworker looked helpless.

It was 12:35.

"Let me check your ears", I said, gesturing with the wall mounted otoscope.

"I can't hear!" the man shouted.

As I leaned toward him I could smell the odor of ear wax. I tried to gently grab and pull his right ear upward and back while I held the otoscope head between my right thumb and index finger and leaned the pinky-side of my hand against his cheek.

His head moved back and forth, up and down. Pushing my right hand firmly into his cheek, I moved with him, as if we were both bouncing on an underinflated air mattress.

All I saw was ear wax.

I repeated the procedure with his left ear. It, too was impacted with black, smelly cerumen.

"Let me flush your ears", I said, loudly, into his right ear.

"I can't hear!" he hollered back.

"I'll be back", I said and gestured with my index finger straight up as in "one minute".

So followed an awkward dance with the man sitting in the exam room chair by the sink, Chux pad on his shoulder, the caseworker holding the cup under his ear and me flushing his right ear with lukewarm water from a large plastic syringe. All three of us moved in near-unison, again and again in what looked like multiple attempts to master a Tango step, sometimes rising at the end, sometimes sinking down or pausing mid-movement, all three of us.

The ear wax poured into the cup and large amounts of water saturated the Chux pad and the side of the man's neck. Some of it landed on me. As I eased myself away each time from our virtual embrace to empty the cup of clumpy wax soup into the sink, I watched through my splattered glasses for a reaction.

After the fifth or sixth serving, the man's movements stopped suddenly. He shook his head like a wet dog. Slowly, he cocked his head and I could sense how he was trying to listen.

The aura in the room changed. Everything seemed quiet and peaceful. He was perfectly still for what seemed like half a minute. The caseworker picked up her clipboard and clicked her ballpoint pen. The ceiling air vents blew their gentle, artificial breeze. Someone walked down the hall outside the exam room.

"I can hear again. Thank you", he said in a normal voice.

"Fantastic. Are you ready for the other ear?" I gestured with the otoscope. It was 12:49.

His head started to gently move again.

"Let's roll!" he grinned.

48) WHERE DOES IT HURT?

"Noncardiac Chest Pain" was Laurie Black's discharge diagnosis. Her chest CT Angiogram didn't show a pulmonary embolus, her troponins were negative for a heart attack and her nuclear stress test was negative for coronary ischemia.

"So what do you think it was?", she asked while I read through her hospital discharge summary.

"I don't know...show me where the pain was", I answered.

"It started in my back, on the left side, and then it went up and around to the front and then down my left arm and my hand felt kind of tingly."

"Where in your back, upper or lower?"

"Upper."

I palpated her left trapezius and put some pressure between her spine and her scapula.

"I assume the doctors at the hospital did all kinds of poking and prodding here", I asked.

"No, I don't think anybody really touched me", Laurie answered.

"Can you move your shoulders around a bit", I asked as I pushed my fingers in a little harder.

"That's very sore", she said, and I could feel the tightness in her muscle.

I moved to her front and asked her to show me the range of motion in her neck. It seemed close to normal.

"Try to go a little further", I said.

"Ouch, I just felt something, in my arm", she startled.

"Looks like it's all coming from your neck. How about that..."

Just a few days earlier I had another "aha" moment, this one regarding a patient with abdominal pain.

Nora Friedman had seen one of my colleagues with a one month history of a painful lump in her right lower abdomen. She ended up with both a CT scan and an ultrasound, and the only abnormality they showed was a very large cyst in the lower portion of her right kidney. The radiologists suggested this cyst could be drained in order to relieve her pain. That's where I came into the picture and as she is on blood thinners, I ended up fussing with the management of her anticoagulants before and after the procedure.

When I saw her after it was done, she told me that her pain hadn't changed at all.

"Show me where it hurts", I asked her.

"Here", she said and laid her hand across her abdomen near McBurney's point.

I asked her to lie down. She did and I felt nothing.

"I actually feel it more when I stand up", she offered.

As she stood in front of me and I placed my hand where she directed me, I asked her to cough. Suddenly I felt a soft, almost squishy protrusion under my fingers.

I called the interventional radiologist who had aspirated her renal cyst through a long needle in her back. He confirmed that her cyst wasn't likely to have reaccumulated that quickly and I told him that both she and I thought we felt a hernia when she stood up and coughed.

"I'm looking at her CT right now..."

His voice trailed and there was a long silence.

"Actually, I can see a spigelian hernia now. That would explain everything. She needs to see a surgeon."

So, in hindsight, a more carful examination of the patient at our end, and of the images at the radiology end, could have saved Nora an invasive procedure, just like Laurie could have been spared some of her fancy hospital tests for what turned out to be a simple neck problem instead of a cardiovascular emergency.

49) MY NEUROLOGY PROFESSOR'S HEADACHES

He spoke with an aura of superiority, in a slightly nasal voice, and his topic was migraines. It was in the late 70's, a time when there were few options to treat migraines.

"Most people who claim to have migraines just have simple tension headaches", he scoffed. And in a move that seemed unorthodox at the time, he disclosed that he himself suffered from "real migraines", so he knew all about this exclusive disease. He made it sound almost desirable by virtue of how rare it was.

At a Continuing Medical Education course in Boston twenty five years ago, I heard a different neurologist, this one a Dutchman, pronounce that most headaches are in fact migraines.

Today I read in The New York Times that, according to a study (published in Headache fourteen years ago) "primary care providers who diagnose a patient's headaches as something other than migraine were usually wrong".

The same article also points out that "sinus headaches" are not a medical reality, and are never diagnosed in Europe. Now that I think of it, I never did hear about this type of headache until I came here.

The whole notion that one explanation for a symptom is somehow more prestigious than another is bizarre, but I see this phenomenon here and there. Also, Americans seem to delight in using technical diagnostic terms instead of describing symptoms to each other or their doctors.

People come into my office all the time with "colitis", "vertigo", "eczema" or "bronchitis", not just diarrhea, dizziness, rashes or coughs. It's like somehow they don't need me to do anything except release my power and prescribe for the condition they already know they have. Never mind that the real explanation may be giardiasis, a cerebellar stroke, psoriasis or lung cancer.

One of the reasons for the seemingly increasing prevalence of certain disease is, of course, the drug company ads for medications that come to market for rare or previously untreatable conditions.

Ironically, as an example of that, back at Uppsala University, I remember a cursory mention of Restless Leg Syndrome. "You can prescribe a little diazepam, that usually helps", was the take-home message. Nobody mentioned that our own neurology professor, Karl-Axel Ekbom, who had retired he same year I started medical school, had described the syndrome, which had been alluded to by Willis in the 1600's, and nobody seemed to make much of its association with iron deficiency.

It was with the introduction of medications like Mirapex and Requip that RLS rose from obscurity to everyday parlance.

Over the past few months I have encountered several patients who, even though they knew they had migraines, had never sought or been offered preventive treatment. There is much awareness of the many medications that treat attacks, and several of those have been cash cows for the pharmaceutical industry, whereas the preventative medications are generally old and inexpensive generics, which require patience and persistence to work.

With many diseases, and very much so with migraines, knowing the diagnosis and the names of some famous medications to treat it is not enough. How to select and titrate them is what we call the Art of Medicine.

50) A NEGATIVE STRESS TEST

Doris Delaney came from the next town. She had just turned sixty and she was worried. For two years she had suffered from chest pain after hard physical work and for the past month her attacks had been a little more frequent.

Her father had died from a heart attack at age 47. Her two brothers had bypass operations before age fifty. Her blood pressure was higher than ideal, even on medication. I flipped through the medical records that had come over on the fax machine and saw that her last LDL cholesterol, on medication, was too high for a high-risk patient.

"I looked on the Internet and I talked to my sister, who is a nurse in Houston. I think I've got angina and I'm worried I've got a blockage in one of my coronary arteries", she said in her thick Texas accent.

I found a two-year-old stress test among the faxed pages and mumbled "I see you had a stress test a while back".

"Yes, and the lady doctor who gave me the stress test told me to go home and take it really easy until I saw my Family Doctor, but he said the test came out okay", she explained.

The first page of the stress test report was the interpretation of the Sestamibi®, or nuclear scan, where a radioactive tracer injected into the bloodstream shows how evenly the blood is distributed between various parts of the heart muscle at rest and with exercise. "Probably normal" was the conclusion rendered by the offsite cardiologist who interpreted the images.

The second page was the report of what the physician saw when Doris did her treadmill exercise test. It said she had chest pain for several minutes at the end of the test and changes on her electrocardiogram that were fairly typical for ischemia, decreased blood flow to the heart muscle.

"I know what happened", I told her.

"A hundred years ago we would diagnose somebody with heart disease by listening to their story. Someone with your symptoms was said to have angina pectoris", I explained.

"When I was in medical school we did EKG stress tests, and they were pretty good at identifying patients with partially blocked arteries. The EKG waveform changes when the heart muscle is stressed, because electricity travels differently through it.

The modern nuclear scan measures something a little different, not whether the muscle is feeling the lack of blood flow but how much blood we see in the picture going to each part of the heart. We think the nuclear test is more sensitive than the EKG, but I don't know that it always is.

In your case you have symptoms that are very suspicious for having blocked arteries, and one part of your stress test was abnormal. Now you are having chest pain more often, and I want you to see a cardiologist as soon as possible. I think they will want to do a catheterization to look at your coronary arteries.

Today I need to give you a prescription for nitroglycerin, change your cholesterol medication and start you on one more blood pressure medication. These three things can make a difference right away."

I had her wait in the room for a few minutes while I called the cardiology office at Cityside Hospital and spoke with Dr. Bronwen Wilkes about getting a fast-track consultation. It's all set; her appointment is Monday.

51) INSIDE AND OUT

77 year old Edward Tripp had been to the emergency room with chest pain last Friday night. It was relentless, aching, and involved the upper part of his left chest.

He had no cough, fever or shortness of breath. He was not sweaty or nauseous, and his blood work, EKG and chest X-ray were normal. He was distinctly tender over the part of his rib cage where bone and cartilage join each other a few inches from his breastbone. He had indeed done some heavy work with his arms in the days before, so the doctor made the assessment that his pain was caused by this apparent costochondritis.

Ed received a shot of pain medication at the hospital and was sent home with a prescription for hydrocodone. As the weekend went by, he started to feel worse and worse.

When I saw him Monday morning, he looked pale. He was short of breath and lightheaded. He had no appetite, and he had been sweating with the slightest exertion.

His blood pressure was low, even for him, a tall, sinewy vegetarian, and his pulse was 115. He did not have a fever, and his oxygen saturation was normal. On exam, there was no heart murmur and his lungs were clear, but his breath sounds seemed a little weaker on the left. His abdomen was diffusely tender, and he was still quite tender over each rib in the upper part of his left rib cage.

His EKG had some very nonspecific changes, which could conceivably go along with impaired blood flow to his left ventricle. Putting all this together, I recommended that we send him back to the hospital for reevaluation. I wondered about angina, a blood clot in his lungs or internal bleeding in his abdomen. His chest wall strain was clearly not the only thing going on.

At the hospital, they did another chest X-ray, which showed some minimal haziness in the left lung. His cardiac enzymes were normal, but he had an elevated D-dimer, so there was a possibility that he had a blood clot in his lung.

His CT angiogram ruled out a clot, but he had a dense infiltrate, by all indications a pneumonia, in his left upper lung, exactly underneath his sore ribs.

When the first chest X-ray was re-read with the second one and the CT as comparisons, the pneumonia was faintly visible.

We all tend to look for one diagnosis that explains everything that is going on with the patient, and we often tend to latch on to the first positive finding we make. But medicine is often more complicated than that, and sometimes we see diseases in early stages, when findings are too subtle to make a diagnosis.

I have come to feel a certain discomfort deep in my gut when an older patient has pain in or even near the chest that appears to have an orthopedic cause.

That feeling dates back to my first job, just out of residency, when an 80 year old woman with shoulder pain I had evaluated came back to the emergency room two hours later with an obvious myocardial infarction on her EKG.

Being the first one to evaluate a patient, you don't have the advantage of elapsed time that the second examiner has. Such is primary and emergency care.

52) THE GREAT IMPOSTER

"I hate to leave you with such an unfinished workup", my senior colleague, Dr. Wilford Brown, said three Thursdays ago. He was going on vacation and Norman Sprague had just been in to see him with a one day history of a strange pain near his right shoulder blade.

Mr. Sprague is a 68 year old retired accountant with rheumatism and diabetes. Dr. Brown ordered some bloodwork and a chest X-ray and told the patient to stay in touch with me about his symptoms.

"I wonder if it's early shingles", Dr. Brown told me.

The next day I got the negative wet read of the chest X-ray and a bunch of normal blood tests and a phone message from Mr. Sprague that he was getting some nausea. I told Autumn to have him come in to get reexamined.

Norman didn't have a fever, and he didn't have a rash or any alteration of skin sensation on his torso. His lymph nodes and breath sounds were normal and his abdomen was soft. But if I pressed hard enough over his gallbladder, he did hurt - that was obvious from his facial expression. He told me the pain was also I the lower front of his chest now, to the right of his sternum just by his lowest rib. It was relentlessly steady and unaffected by movements or deep breathing. He denied any shortness of breath. He told me was nauseous but still able to eat a little, and he had not vomited. His ribs weren't tender. His bowels were normal and his urine had normal color.

I ordered a gallbladder ultrasound. There were no gallstones, but the radiologist said there was a suggestion of sludge in the gallbladder and the common bile duct was at the upper limit of normal size.

I called one of our local surgeons. He suggested doing a plain HIDA scan. Because of the national shortage of cholecystokinin, that is the only type of biliary scan we can get right now. The test showed that the gallbladder filled normally, but the tracer was slow to travel down the bile ducts and into the duodenum.

Last Monday, Norman met with the surgeon, who called and said he was pretty sure the pain was biliary, but also told me that over the weekend before the consultation, Norman had developed shortness of breath and dizziness. I asked him to send Norman over so I could reassess him.

He was not all that short of breath and did not have a cough, but his breathing had changed since I saw him last. He admitted that he had had some difficulty shopping at Walmart since last winter because he felt "out of shape" pushing a cart up and down the aisles. He also described his right-sided chest pain as more severe, but still unrelated to movement and breathing.

He had dizziness and a hint of nystagmus only when turning his head to the left in a supine position with an otherwise normal ENT and neuro exam, so I was comfortable ascribing his dizziness to Benign Positional Vertigo.

His oxygen saturation was normal and his EKG was unchanged from three years ago.

I ordered a PE protocol contrast chest CT, which did not show any pulmonary emboli, but it did show mildly enlarged mediastinal lymph nodes and three nodules peripherally in the right lung, the largest one just over an inch. I had also ordered an abdominal CT, which was perfectly normal. The nuclear stress test I also ordered that day came back normal. By that time I had called Cityside Pulmonary Associates. They promised to look over the images and get back to us with an appointment.

Norman Sprague called back two days later. He had received a call from the pulmonary office, telling him he was on a cancellation list, but only had a firm appointment for the first week in October.

I called the thoracic surgery group at Cityside and got to talk with Dan Grossman. He looked at the images and when I asked him if a video assisted thoracoscopy was an option for getting a tissue diagnosis, he said, yes, but bronchoscopy would be better. I told him about the long want to see a pulmonologist.

"Either we or they will see him sooner", Dan said. I'll get back to you. Twenty minutes later he called me back. "It's all set, Roger White will see him on Friday and do a scope then."

Norman had his bronchoscopy. The needle aspirates were benign and the washings and cultures negative. Dr. White's note listed sarcoidosis and methotrexate related lung disease as the top differential diagnoses, and he thought a PET CT would be the next step, and maybe a percutaneous needle biopsy of the distal lesions.

Today I met with Norman and his wife to go over the results that had come in after the bronchoscopy. As I reexamined his abdomen, he was more tender in the right upper quadrant than before, and when I lifted up the back of his shirt there was a red spot with a small, raised center, not a blister but more of a papule.

"Ouch, that's sore", he said.

And so I leave Norman Sprague in the competent hands of Dr. Brown, who returns from his vacation tomorrow. Norman's lung nodules and lymphadenopathy still remain to be diagnosed, and he still may have gallbladder disease, but he also, again, has the original working diagnosis of herpes zoster, the great imposter.

53) AN ACT TO END CONSTIPATION

I never contemplated bananas very much until the other day, after I counseled a patient with diarrhea about the BRAT diet, consisting of bananas, rice, applesauce and toast. The next two patients I saw were in their 80's, on fluid pills and bothered by constipation. Both patients were eating at least one banana per day for fear of low potassium.

Since that day I have informally polled constipated patients about their breakfast habits. My early results suggest that more constipated patients have cereal with milk and banana for breakfast than their non-constipated peers.

Many processed grains, particularly wheat, can be constipating. Dairy products are also constipating for many people. But bananas, fruits with lots of fiber, are they also constipating?

Reading what scientific literature I was able to find on the subject of bananas and constipation, I found several mentions of a theory that unripe, starchy, bananas are constipating, whereas ripe bananas promote regularity.

The obvious next phase of my inquiry will be to ask my banana eating patients how they prefer their bananas, ripe or more "al dente". I know that whenever I look at bananas in the store, too many black spots on the skin makes me think they're about to go bad, and I prefer the less sweet taste of what might be considered unripe bananas.

When I lived in Sweden, I saw a little less constipation than here, so it was a surprise to me when I read that the Swedes eat more bananas than other westerners. I know for a fact that extra ripe bananas are not preferred there. My theory on why the Swedes aren't plagued by constipation to match their banana consumption is that they are more physically active, even into old age, than Americans. In my mother's neighborhood, she and many other octogenarians were always out with their rolling walkers, going to the store, the bus stop or just taking a stroll.

I am beginning to formulate a better, more pragmatic approach to geriatric constipation now that I have become aware of the dichotomy of bananas. Of course, I have to also be more diligent in dispelling the myth that everybody on fluid pills has to eat a banana a day.

Another aspect of adult and geriatric constipation I have become more and more aware of is that many people with constipation get worse by eating high fiber foods. Patients with bulky, hard stools can get even bulkier stools from extra fiber. For such patients, high fiber breakfast cereal with milk and unripe banana is the ultimate insult to regularity, and a habit to be discouraged.

An apple a day may keep the doctor away as whole apples relieve constipation.

A banana a day, on the other hand, may bring about more business for the doctor.

54) CLARA'S SINUS HEADACHES

When people come to my office with "sinus headaches", they often ask for an antibiotic and perhaps something for congestion. Pain in the forehead, behind the eyes or in the cheekbone area doesn't always mean infection, though.

Clara was a widow in her seventies, who had experienced frequent and severe sinus headaches for years. She even had postnasal drip and a recurrent sore throat. I ordered a CT scan, which was negative; there was no sign of cancer or polyps, but also no sign of sinusitis. On this, one of many office visits, she asked for antibiotics. I agreed to prescribe something while we waited to get the scan.

When we had a follow-up visit to review the scan, I told her the films were completely normal. She told me the antibiotics had cleared all her symptoms, just like every time her previous doctor had prescribed them. How could she not have had a sinus infection when the antibiotics always made her feel better? It wasn't long before she came back with another request for antibiotics.

The antibiotics always had to be brand name - she insisted generics made her feel badly and they never cleared her sinuses. The pharmacists would point out that the generic version of her favorite antibiotic was actually made by the same manufacturer as the brand name. Clara was unconvinced. She had good insurance, and all she needed me to do was check the box on the prescription and write "Brand Medically Necessary". This is what she insisted on for her antibiotics as well as for her maintenance heart medications.

I didn't feel comfortable with Clara's repeated requests for antibiotics, so I sent her for a couple more CT scans over the years, and she reluctantly agreed to see an allergist and an ear, nose and throat specialist. She didn't like either of them, and they didn't help her. She seemed to enjoy her visits with me, and she often said that she wouldn't know what to do without me; on the way out she would hug me good-bye.

Clara often seemed a little sad and lost. Her husband had always taken good care of her, although I wasn't sure how happy their marriage had been. She had never involved herself with practical or financial matters. Now she was struggling with what to do with their mobile home in Florida, and she fretted about whether to sell their house, which was too large and too expensive to heat. I would try to help her find the confidence to tackle things one at a time.

We finally had a heart-to-heart talk about her headaches. I suggested we stop treating her with antibiotics, and she asked me if I thought she was just imagining them. I reassured her that I didn't think so, but explained that you can have temporary congestion without infection.

Clara sold her home and moved into a senior citizen complex. I was busy, and didn't notice how much time had passed. One day recently my office nurse, Autumn, grinned and said "Guess who just made an appointment to switch all her prescriptions to generics!"

Clara entered the office with an air of confidence and dressed to the nines. "You look well", I pointed out. "I'm happy," she beamed, and pointed out a new diamond ring.

Clara had not been in for well over six months. She never had headaches anymore, and she thought it was time she tried the generics. I knew her problem had never been her sinuses. And I knew it wasn't all in her head; all along it had been in her heart.

55) OPIATES, PAIN AND INTEGRATION

We are witnessing a strange migration of restless tribes, moving between doctors and clinics, traveling great distances in search of what no one wants to give them anymore.

This eerie movement is steadily gaining momentum in our community, in our state and across the country. We can hear it in telephone calls, we can read it in records of patients looking to switch their care, and we can see it in the eyes of the hopefuls who hobble through our doors, looking for a doctor who will contradict their previous provider and reinstate the status quo: a steady supply of opioids for their pain.

The CDC has made new recommendations for opiate dosing and monitoring, and our state is legislating finite opioid dosing limits. Colleagues everywhere are tapering doses, scouring new and existing patients' prescription monitoring reports, and aggressively enforcing their opioid contracts by doing more urine drug screens and pill counts than in the past.

Last week, two new patients no-showed for their first appointment after the intake nurse called them to make sure they were aware of our prescription policies. Yesterday, a new patient I sent home the day before to bring me her most recent oxycodone pill bottle called back saying it was empty. It shouldn't have been. I offered to take care of her other medical needs but I let her know I would not be prescribing narcotics for her. I doubt she'll be making the 45 minute trip again.

Most of the people I see looking for a new source of pain medications are of the baby boomer generation, grandparents and even retirees, and have been diagnosed with lumbar disc disease. Many carry the diagnosis of fibromyalgia, and almost all of them report symptoms of depression, anxiety and PTSD.

I also see a surprising number of adults with a diagnosis of attention deficit disorder, who have been cut off their prescribed stimulant medications. They were diagnosed as middle aged adults, not during their school years.

Most of these medical migrants seem to be singularly focused on finding a source for the prescriptions they have relied on for many years. Only a few, like the grandmotherly sixty eight year old woman I saw yesterday, say they want to manage their chronic pain and are willing to hear what options I can offer them. This woman had a large hole in her nasal septum from snorting cocaine decades earlier.

This particular woman told me that a month after she was cut off from her opioids, she actually had a three or four week stretch when she hardly felt any pain at all. Then, gradually, her pain returned. She didn't have any idea of what made it go away and then return.

I told her she had just experienced the power of her own mind over the vicious cycle of sensory input and faulty interpretation of its significance. She eagerly accepted my offer to enroll in our pain management program that day.

She is one of the few new or prospective patients I have met lately who told me she wanted to experience less pain, rather than get a certain prescription.

Pain is a mysterious phenomenon. Our four session pain program, offered individually and not in groups, helps patients understand how pain perceptions work, and gives them a sense of control they never had before. Many participants voluntarily reduce their dose of pain medications after attending, and a large proportion of those on low doses get off them completely.

I introduce the basic idea behind the classes by telling my patients about an old Boy Scout trick:

Sitting by the campfire, you put a branding iron in with the embers and watch it get glowing hot. Then you blindfold the newest member of the troop and expose his arm. While you place the branding iron on a slab of bacon, making it smoke and sizzle, you touch the person's bare arm with a smuggled-in Popsicle.

What sensation does the poor newcomer experience? Cold or heat?

The answer is intense heat, 99% of the time.

Pain exists in the brain, where noxious stimuli from our bodies are given meaning. The idea, and it is a vey powerful one, is that we can learn to change our interpretation of our own noxious stimuli. They are only nerve signals. Our minds, through our past experiences and because of our expectations, can change their character, intensity and significance.

Opioids do nothing to our aching backs, knees or feet; they just create a certain level of more or less modest euphoria that helps us reframe the meaning of unwanted nerve signals from our arthritic joints.

And now the pendulum is gaining momentum in its swing from one extreme to the other: Pain isn't a vital sign anymore. Opioids aren't safe anymore. They're hardly ever indicated anymore. But we can't just stop them without offering something else. We can offer an empowering understanding of how pain works, and we can help reduce the broader suffering that we used to speak of only in terms of physical pain.

50% of our patients who have completed the pain sessions have asked to continue seeing their behavioral health professional to work on other issues.

By speaking of pain matter-of-factly, we create a platform for also dealing with other kinds of suffering.

This is true integration of behavioral and primary care.

56) "THE FOUR HORSEMEN OF THE MEDICAL APOCALYPSE": IT'S ALL ABOUT INFLAMMATION

"Although there may never be such a single path, mounting evidence suggests a common underlying cause of major degenerative diseases. The four horsemen of the medical apocalypse — coronary artery disease, diabetes, cancer, and Alzheimer's — may be riding the same steed: inflammation."
– Harvard Health Letter, 2006

It has been said that it takes 17 years for new scientific information to change medical practice. So, it's been 14 years since Harvard posted the article titled "Inflammation: A unifying theory of disease".

Note the dramatic allegory, "The four horsemen of the medical apocalypse". The chronic diseases listed plus obesity and probably also depression, which is now costing more in disability payments than back pain and other musculoskeletal conditions combined, are driving our healthcare expenses into the stratosphere and our population into a quagmire of suffering and death from diseases that seem to actually be preventable and in many cases reversible.

What is inflammation?

A cut or scrape heals through the process of inflammation, which is a good thing. But too much inflammation can make that process go overboard and a thick, raised keloid scar forms.

Pounding your heels on a concrete factory floor day after day can cause mechanical stress on the plantar fascia, the tendon-like band that helps maintain the arch of your foot.

Through the process of inflammation, part of that fascia undergoes thickening and eventually calcification, and a heel spur forms.

A ruptured disc in your lower back can cause acute pressure on the nerves that supply feeling and control muscle activity in your leg – sciatica. In response to this pressure, the injured nerve swells through the process of inflammation and becomes even more squeezed than it was from the initial injury.

Chronic disc problems can cause calcification, just like with heel spurs, at the corners of each vertebra and sharp bone spurs can form in your back.

Autoimmune diseases like arthritis, psoriasis and colitis involve similar processes in our bodies. Misguided efforts to repair minimal or imaginary (on the part of the immune system) damage or fight off "foreign" invasion cause changes to our bodies like bone spurs or destruction, rashes or peeling skin and diarrhea or ulcer formation, and profound alterations in mood and cognitive ability.

Inflammation can also occur inside our blood vessels. It is now well known that foods and chemicals can increase or decrease inflammation, which helps determine whether blood borne fats start building up in the walls of our blood vessels.

More and more evidence also implicates inflammation as a contributor to obesity , which in turn can promote more inflammation.

The new movement of Functional Medicine is studying and promoting non-pharmaceutical approaches to these inflammation mediated medical conditions. Calling their philosophy "The medicine of why", they reject the idea that the best way to fight inflammatory diseases is by suppressing the immune system. Instead they focus on avoiding triggers, correcting deficiencies and reversing the modern day imbalance between helpful and excessive immune responses. I have written about this before, here.

The frighteningly simple theory is now more and more anchored in science, down to the specific chemical reactions at work in our bodies and the dietary phytochemicals involved. What we eat, drink, inhale or otherwise expose ourselves to can cause or prevent disease and can determine whether our genetic risks manifest in disease or not. This exploding field is called epigenetics.

How do we fight inflammation?

Here are some very simple fundamentals about what everyone can do to reduce their risk of the inflammation mediated diseases Harvard called the medical apocalypse:

Pro-inflammatory foods to avoid:

Sugar and high fructose corn syrup as well as "refined carbohydrates", which means anything made from flour (bread, pasta, crackers, boxed breakfast cereals and many snack foods).

Artificial trans fats or partially hydrogenated oils (now phased out from our food supply).

So called "tropical" oils like palm and coconut oil.

Processed meats.

Excessive alcohol.

Also, although not foods, inhaled substances like cigarette smoke can cause inflammation and at the same time decrease normal immune defense responses.

<u>Anti-inflammatory foods to choose:</u>

Healthy Omega-3 fats like olive oil, fatty fish like salmon, avocado and tree nuts.

Berries, cherries, grapes and tomatoes.

Vegetables like broccoli, Brussels sprouts and kale.

Turmeric, cocoa and green tea.

(More details here: https://www.healthline.com/nutrition/13-anti-inflammatory-foods)

Of course, there is more, but imagine if everyone took these simple steps – olive oil consumption alone reduces heart attack risk by 25%, for example.

I am still puzzling about why we aren't thinking and talking much more about this. Unfortunately, it seems this is not going to revolutionize medical practice in a mere 17 years.

57) A POSTHUMOUS BLESSING

Mitch Tapley was not your ordinary preacher. He was a burly man in his late sixties with massive, tattoo-covered arms, a stubbly, broad face and hair that always looked like he might have arrived by motorcycle. He smelled of cigarette smoke and his powerful baritone voice had a gravelly edge to it that reminded me of Johnny Cash.

He became my patient just a few months ago after he ended up in the hospital and almost died from a respiratory illness. Mitch had worked hard to get back in the pulpit and out among his congregation, and every time I had seen him he had spoken of trying to find a balance between helping others and taking care of his own health.

Our last visit, the day before yesterday, seemed particularly profound. He spoke of his walk with his Lord by his side, and a new level of clarity he had experienced since facing his own mortality, then interrupted himself and said:

"I don't even know if you are a believer, but I think you know what I mean."

I responded by telling him what my father had said about my choice of medicine as a career many years ago - that I could have been a lawyer but I was too honest, or a preacher but my faith was too weak.

He laughed heartily and said:

"God bless you, man, you are a healer and a friend."

I asked him again about his smoking, and he said he was almost ready to quit.

Early this morning the shrill sound of an ambulance tore through our little village and the news reached me as I walked through the clinic door: Pastor Mitch had suffered a massive heart attack and died from cardiac arrest.

This afternoon I dialed his home number to give my condolences to his wife. The phone rang four or five times, then there was a click, followed by his familiar, powerful, resonant voice. A chill went up my spine as the recording played:

"I am not here to take your call,

Please try again later, and

May the Lord always be with you.

May He bless you and protect you.

May His face smile on you and be gracious to you.

May the Lord show you His favor and give you His peace."

58) SOMETIMES YOU JUST GOTTA TREAT IT

"Red" McDougall had terrible leg pains soon after going to bed. He did have a bad back, and some mild spinal stenosis, but I hadn't heard much about that in the past few years. He was just dealing with the ache in his legs when he was on his feet too long.

A few months ago he saw his vascular surgeon for a routine followup. He'd had a femoral-popliteal bypass to restore circulation to his right leg a few years ago. The vascular surgeon was intrigued by the fact that both legs hurt when elevated. That is usually a sign of severe ischemia, but Red's pulses were palpable. To play it safe, the surgeon ordered formal pulse volume recordings and a CT angiogram.

The studies were normal and the surgeon speculated that the pain could be related to Red's bad back.

I saw him for a diabetes followup a few weeks ago. He had ever so slightly decreased monofilament sensation in both feet and his legs had normal strength, normal reflexes and no atrophy.

"Does it feel like cramps?" I asked.

"Not really, they just hurt", Red answered. "It's so bad I have to sit on the edge of my bed and dangle my legs or walk around a bit before it goes away. But it's driving me crazy. I hardly get any sleep anymore."

"Well, we know it's not your circulation", I began. "It could be just a form of leg cramps, even though you can't tell if there is spasm in the muscles. Or it could be a strange way for your spinal stenosis to act up in the opposite position from the way it usually behaves. So I have an idea."

"Anything", he was quick to answer.

"Cyclobenzaprine. A muscle relaxer that is related to the antidepressant amitriptyline. In addition to preventing muscle spasms, it has pain relieving properties and it usually helps people sleep."

"Gimme some", Red held out his hand.

"I'll send in a script. Let me see you back in two weeks, because if this doesn't work, I'll need to do some serious thinking."

I thought to myself about how often specialists are in a position where they can simply declare "Not my department", but primary care docs are then more or less obligated to pick up the ball again and do something.

Two weeks later, Red was a new man.

I'm sleeping through the night, and no pain", he grinned.

I still don't know exactly what this was, but it's gone.

Sometimes you just gotta treat it.

59) AN ACCIDENTAL CURE

I have one patient in each of my clinics with a long history of relentless abdominal pain, mild constipation, poor appetite and general malaise. Neither one has any abnormality on any of the testing I or my colleagues at the clinic or in the nearest hospital have done: An alphabet soup of blood tests, CT scans, ultrasounds, endoscopies, gastric emptying studies and I don't know what.

Each one of these older gentlemen usually comes in looking pale and gaunt, saying "I just don't feel good, Doc".

Now, one of them seems to be cured, within three days of starting a new prescription, intended to treat something else.

Hector Dunn happened to come in with a COPD exacerbation within a couple of months of his last one. I prescribed the usual steroid, but, because it hadn't been too long since he had taken the usual Bactrim, I put him on doxycycline.

When I saw him in followup, my medical assistant warned me: "You're not going to believe this, but Hector looks and feels like a million bucks".

I knocked on the door of his exam room and entered.

He jumped out of his seat, grinned and gave me a strong, firm handshake.

"I feel better than I've felt in years after that last prescription. My breathing got better right away, but my stomach feels great, I don't hurt anywhere and I have all kinds of energy. I'd say I feel the best I have felt in twenty years."

His wife nodded and chimed in:

"The day after he started the doxycycline, he got rid of all kinds of gas over about 48 hours, and then he was like a new man."

I sat quietly and took in the scene before my eyes and, just like with the patient I once had hat developed Parkinson's disease under my nose and was diagnosed and treated by someone else, I suddenly saw Hector move his face while he talked, shift forward in his chair, make gestures with his hands, arms and shoulders as he provided more vivid and extraneous details about his colonic gas elimination. I had never seen him that lively; before that, he had always carried himself as if any extra effort or movement might cause him to crump.

"Could that antibiotic have gotten rid of some intestinal infection he had been carrying for years", his wife asked, astutely.

"Absolutely", I answered. "It's called SIBO, or Small Intestine Bacterial Overgrowth. While we are supposed to have billions of bacteria in our large intestine, the small intestine should not have bacteria in it. Sometimes it does, and that can cause anything from diarrhea to chronic abdominal pain and bloating, and I now have to admit that may have been what Mr. Dunn has had for a long time now. There's no handy test for it so sometimes we just guess and treat, but it had not occurred to me. Doxycycline isn't the typical treatment for it, but it can work, and doxycycline also has some antiinflammatory properties, and SIBO may have elements of inflammation linked to it."

"I don't know what any of that really means, but I do know I feel good", Hector concluded, rose from his chair and patted me on the shoulder. He seemed eager to get out of there, unlike other times when I was probably the one who wanted the visit to end because of my own helplessness.

"Now, I'll need to hear if the belly pain comes back", I said. If it does, we'll have to decide if we're going to use doxycycline again, or the stuff the books say might work even better. Let me know how you're doing, okay?"

146

Later that day, I thought about my other patient, Percy Barr. What if he might respond to doxycycline, too? But he's on warfarin, and there's an interaction between those two drugs. I'd probably give him rifaximin. But he's in Florida, as every other winter.

So in a twist of fate, I'm starting to look forward to him coming back, now that I have something different, new and promising to offer him.

60) NOT ON CALL

"I am not on call", Dr. Brian Stoltz said over a lot of background noise through what must have been the speakerphone in his car.

"I know", I said. "Cityside ER said there is nobody on call for ophthalmology this weekend. I have a 54 year old woman with intense tearing, discomfort and only 20/70 vision in her right eye."

"And she's not a patient of our office?"

"No, she has only had to see an optometrist for glasses. I've called every hospital within 50 miles and there is no ophthalmologist on call over the long weekend. You helped me once before with a case of dendritic keratitis when you were on call."

I also remembered Memorial Day weekend last year, I was in the same situation during my Saturday clinic. A young boy, whose mother had just joined the board of our health center, came in with eye irritation. He had a small rust ring very close to the center of his cornea. I had dug out plenty of them, with a special spatula or even with the tip of an 18 gauge needle, but this was a child, who might not have been fully cooperative, and the location was critical for his future near vision.

Cityside Hospital had no ophthalmologist on call for that long weekend either, and all my calls to ophthalmologists in the surrounding area were fruitless. He got in to see an eye doctor the Wednesday after the Monday holiday and it turned out that he actually also had a small metallic corneal foreign body. Everything turned out okay, but the wait was uncomfortable and at least a little risky.

A corneal rust ring, even a foreign body, can usually wait a few days, but if this woman had what I thought, acute angle closure glaucoma, I wouldn't want her to wait that long to see an eye doctor.

"I think she's got acute glaucoma", I said.

He was silent. I continued:

"She's got mixed injection, no foreign body, no fluorescein uptake and I can see her left fundus clearly but I can't get a focus on her right fundus no matter what lens I dial in on the ophthalmoscope."

He was silent again for what seemed a very long time. Then he said:

"I live an hour away, but I happen to be in town. If you have her walk out your door right now, I'll meet her at my office in, what, 25 minutes?"

"She'll be there. Thank you so much."

I haven't heard yet what he found, and I haven't wanted to bug him, but I am anxious to hear what the final diagnosis was. I do know that an urgent slit lamp exam was necessary.

One postscript:

When I sent my emergency eye patient off with her office note and insurance information to see Dr. Stoltz, her husband said:

"You've done well by us. I came in and saw you once with a cauda equina syndrome."

I didn't remember him, but he must have had a critical enough pressure on his lower spinal nerves to also have warranted an urgent referral to a specialist.

Disease strikes at inopportune times.

61) EXIT DIAGNOSIS

Dwayne Tarlov came to see me today for pain in his right wrist and left ankle for the past month and a half.

There hadn't been much swelling, and he had no morning stiffness to suggest rheumatism. He had not had any fever or cold symptoms, and he absolutely denied any injury or new activities that might have brought on his symptoms.

His exam revealed his usual habitus, a slender, fine-boned fifty five year old man with gray hair, a tightly cropped beard and a new stud earring in his left ear.

His right wrist had normal range of movement, but localized swelling and tenderness near the extensor tendons of his thumb. There was no clicking or catching with thumb movements and I felt no crepitations.

The ankle was puffy on the outer, lateral, side and Dwayne was a little tender. Turning his ankle outward was painful.

I ordered X-rays, prescribed ibuprofen and recommended a wrist splint. We agreed to see how he is doing in two weeks. I asked again, and Dwayne could not remember anything he could have done to cause his pains.

I went back to my office to check messages and touch base with Autumn. A few moments later I was startled by a loud motor exhaust. Looking out the window, I saw Dwayne on a large Harley-Davidson motorcycle. His right wrist revved the gas, he squeezed the clutch and with his left foot, he kicked the bike into gear and roared off across the parking lot.

I typed an addendum to his office note to remind me about my exit diagnosis of his wrist and ankle pain.

62) NEVER ASSUME

Peter Bartley came into the office today with a two day history of black, tarry stools. The day before this started, he had had a terrible case of indigestion and took several slugs of Pepto-Bismol to quiet it down. This had helped, and he was feeling quite well today, but the color of his stools bothered him.

"His stools are probably black because of the Pepto", Autumn said as she filled me in. I had another patient to see before Peter, so I asked Autumn to get orthostatic vitals on him while I went in to see Norma Daigle for her regular 3 month visit.

Norma's thyroid test was normal, and her blood pressure was stable, but she looked very concerned, and she was clutching a pill bottle between her hands.

"Bigtown Pharmacy delivered this yesterday along with my other medicines, but I don't know what it was for, so I didn't take it", she said, adding "there was also a bottle of trazodone, and I took one of those because I used to take them and I knew it worked good helping me sleep".

I looked at the bottle. It contained escitalopram, the generic form of Lexapro. Norma is on lithium and Prozac. Lexapro in addition would be redundant and could cause nausea, heart palpitations and high blood pressure or bring on a manic episode if she were to take it for any length of time. At the upper right hand corner of the label was the prescriber's name, a psychiatrist at Cityside Hospital.

"It's from Dr. Hirsh, did you ever see him?" I handed the bottle back to her. She frowned and said "never heard of him".

I called Bigtown Pharmacy on my cell phone. I posed my question and was put on hold for less than a minute. The pharmacist came on and admitted they had made a mistake. The medication was for Nancy Daigle, another patient of mine.

The pharmacist asked "Can we pick the medications up at your office this afternoon?"

"Well, one bottle is here and the other one is at the patient's house", I explained.

"Tell her we'll pick both up at her house", said the embarrassed pharmacist.

"Good thing you read labels", I said to Norma, who just sat there, shaking her head.

Peter Bartley's standing blood pressure was the same as when he sat down. His pulse was normal. As I placed my hand in the upper center of his abdomen and pushed slowly downward, he winced a little. His black stool tested strongly positive for blood. I told him it looked like he might have a bleeding ulcer and not just black stool from Pepto-Bismol.

My next patient, Beatrice Nash, was in for pain in her left hip. She had already been to the emergency room for this, and her hip x-ray had been normal. As I listened to her symptoms, I knew this was no ordinary groin pull, as the emergency room doctor had thought.

"I hurt more after I stand for a while", Beatrice said.

"Show me where", I asked her, and she put her left hand over the bony pelvis, well above the hip joint. Both hips and both knees had full movement without pain, her straight leg raising test was normal, there was no pain when I resisted her hip movements, and there was no groin hernia when she stood up. After she laid down on the exam table, I palpated her abdomen and there, deep in the left lower quadrant, was a tender mass.

"Is this where you hurt when you stand up", I asked.

"Yes, that's where I hurt", she answered.

"We need to get some bloodwork and a CT scan of your abdomen and pelvis", I said, "because it doesn't look like your hip is the problem. You might have some sort of cyst in your pelvis." I was worried this could be a tumor, but felt pleased that I had come up with a plausible explanation for her pain.

Diane Fehrer's TSH was even more out of range than last time, when I bumped up the dose of her thyroid medicine, and she was feeling very tired.

"Are you sure you haven't missed any pills", I asked her, but she said she was sure she always remembered to take them. "Let me just double check with the pharmacy that you got the right strength", I said and pulled out my cell phone. The pharmacy technician's answers to my questions explained her slipping thyroid status: Diane had not picked up her old dose of levothyroxine for several weeks before her previous blood test, and last months's new prescription was still waiting for her at the drugstore.

Next up was Matt Wikert, who had run some high blood pressures at home. The other day at at the nursing home where he is working as a physical therapist, the nurse had recorded 178/98 and had wondered if I wanted to see him right away. I said to have him check it a few more times and see me today. His pressure at check-in was 148/80.

"So your blood pressure looks better today. How are you feeling", I asked.

"Well, I still have some pressure in my chest...", he began.

My heart sank. The nurse had not said anything about chest pain, and I had not specifically asked. I know better. Fortunately his EKG was normal, and the character of the pain was quite atypical, so it probably isn't angina, but, still, it was a sobering reminder that you really can't assume anything in the practice of medicine:

A chief complaint is often only the patient's self-diagnosis, or interpretation of a symptom. A high blood pressure can seem more significant than a vague pressure in the chest, and a pain above the hip can seem easier to explain as a hip pain than something there is no word for.

A pharmacist or a physician can get their patients mixed up, and patients forget their pills more often than we'd like to believe.

Not all patients with black stool while on Pepto-Bismol have black stool because of the Pepto-Bismol. Some have a bleeding ulcer, which is why they took the Pepto-Bismol in the first place.

And, if we hurry in our work, we are more likely to assume, instead of evaluate and examine thoroughly.

63) NEVER ASSUME - INDEED!

A couple of weeks ago I wrote a post titled "Never Assume" about a handful of patients, whose case histories took an unexpected turn.

Well, as it happened, a few more twists and turns unfolded since then:

Peter Bartley, the man with upper abdominal pain and black stool, not just from the Pepto-Bismol he had taken, had his upper endoscopy. It only showed some mild gastritis without bleeding. Fortunately, the surgeon also did a colonoscopy, which showed an actively bleeding polyp almost the size of a clementine in his transverse colon.

Black stool is generally thought to be from the stomach or duodenum, located above the ligament of Treitz. It has been said that it takes the digestive juices 14 hours to change the color of our hemoglobin into black melena. Peter's intestinal transit time must have been slower than most people's for this to happen with a bleeding polyp in his colon.

Norma Daigle, who had received another patient's trazodone and Lexapro, called the other day and told Autumn she wanted some trazodone of her own, because it had made her sleep so well.

Beatrice Nash, whose hip pain seemed to come from a mass in her left pelvis, had her CT scan. It showed a very large probable lipoma, a harmless fatty tumor. She has seen the surgeon, who wrote in his note that she described the pain as sharp and coming directly from the hip, and not at all from somewhere higher up than that. He didn't think the lipoma had anything to do with the hip pain, and recommended she see an orthopedic surgeon.

As it happened, a few days later she had a follow up visit with her orthopedist for a cortisone shot to her arthritic knee. I eagerly read through his note to see if he thought her pain was from the hip joint or not, but there was no mention at all of her hip pain!

Diane Fehrer, who never seemed to remember to take her thyroid medication, accepted the pharmacy's offer to put her pills in monthly calendar bubble packs. I am keeping my fingers crossed that she will remember to look at the bubble pack every day, and I keep wondering: If she does take her levothyroxine every day, will my prescribed dose be too high and cause her tremors, palpitations or even atrial fibrillation?

Finally, Matt Wikert, the physical therapist with high blood pressure and chest pains, showed up at the hospital for his stress test as planned. Earlier that morning he had a 45 minute episode of chest pain. His EKG showed some subtle changes from the one I had done, so the stress test was cancelled and he was admitted for observation. He ruled out for myocardial infarction and was discharged with plans for a rescheduled stress test. We still don't have a date for it.

Every day, just like that day a few weeks ago, I see patients whose stories don't quite fit the expected pattern. In the words of Sir William Osler:

"Variability is the law of life, and as no two faces are the same, so no two bodies are alike, and no two individuals react alike and behave alike under the abnormal conditions which we know as disease."

64) ADVERSE EFFECTS

Doctors hate it when patients say: "Doc, I don't want to take this medicine, because it causes all these side effects - just look at this list I got from the pharmacist (or off the internet)."

As allopathic physicians, we are at a disadvantage because our medicines come with warnings about every side effect ever reported, even if no one has ever proven it was actually caused by the medication.

Everyone knows about the placebo effect, the healing caused by a patient's expectation that a medication will work. The package inserts we get today bring on the nocebo effect, which is the creation of discomfort by negative expectations.

Practitioners of alternative medicine have it easy; they can take full advantage of the placebo effect without the nocebo effect caused by pharmacists, the FDA, the legal climate or the Internet.

Adverse effects can be very real and frightening, though. I have seen plenty of them, and it does make me careful. This is the age of information and Informed Consent, and we have to be very careful to tell patients about possible adverse effects when we prescribe.

I have seen a woman's bone marrow almost shut down from a week of sulfa for a urinary tract infection. One man lost the use of his right arm for months due to rotator cuff inflammation after taking Cipro for a sinus infection. Another man developed horrendous sunburn while taking doxycycline for a prostate infection. Several patients have developed allergic rashes and tongue swelling.

I have seen people go into heart failure from Avandia, a once-popular diabetes medicine and I have seen people use my prescriptions to try to do themselves in.

But adverse effects can be caused by non-pharmacological treatments also. Sometimes a doctor's words or demeanor can have unintended, even devastating effects.

One successful business woman told me once that she had felt terrible the whole time between two appointments because she had got the impression I thought she was foolish, and I couldn't even remember what had happened. A few times I have had to undo damage I caused by being in a hurry when dealing with a patient who was afraid or anxious.

A physician's demeanor is part of the treatment. I know they teach empathy in medical school these days - to the extent this is something that can be taught.

William Sykes was told by his pulmonologist that he had eighteen months to live when he was diagnosed with alpha-1-antitrypsin deficiency. He became severely depressed. The antidepressants and steroids I prescribed made him manic for a while, but we got through it. I promised him the pulmonologist didn't really know how long he would live. The specialist did fire William as a patient because he cancelled a couple of follow-up appointments, so it was "him and me" and the occasional Hospitalist for a few days of "pulmonary toilet".

William lived almost ten years longer than predicted, even got married and adopted an old parrot, which learned to imitate the sound of the oxygen truck backing into the driveway. But he never got over the words of the pulmonologist.

65) A NEAR MISS, TECHNOLOGY NOTWITHSTANDING

The other day I ordered a CT scan with contrast on a patient with an apparent mass on his neck. I explained about the need to get a blood test to make sure his kidneys could handle the iodine contrast. Because our lab was closed, I had to print a requisition for him to bring to the hospital lab.

Printing a requisition from our EMR is a multi step process that involves leaving the "superbill" (I don't know what's so superior about it, but that's a different topic), going to "chart", clicking on "requisitions", highlighting the "creatinine" I just ordered, selecting "in-house lab" even though the requisition is meant to bring to the hospital, selecting "ok", then getting transported to another screen where I must again highlight "creatinine", clicking "print", getting to a pop up window that says "could not find a printer...", clicking on the name of the only printer on the network I ever use (immediately to the left of my desk back in my office), clicking "ok" and walking back to my office to get the piece of paper, signing it by hand even though it says "electronically signed" and (finally) giving it to the patient.

The next day we got a fax from the x-Ray department with their premedication protocol for iodine allergic patients. I had missed the fact that my patient had an allergy to iodine.

I simply missed the fact that my patient had this allergy, and he didn't catch my comment about "iodine contrast". I should have asked more specifically about iodine allergy, and I should have made the detour from "superbill" to "medications" to "allergies" before going to "chart" to go through the steps of ordering the creatinine, but this time I didn't.

My million dollar system, which doesn't even have a spell checker, doesn't know that a CT with contrast requires a creatinine and is contraindicated if the patient is allergic to iodine. It makes me follow a "workflow" that reminds me of my High School introduction, in the early seventies, to the early programming languages of the day (COBOL and Fortran, if I remember correctly) and my first Atari home computer. It is far removed from the $500 iPhone I carry on my belt.

In the days before our EMR, filling out a paper requisition took only a few seconds and gave me more time and mental space to chat with the patient about the test itself while I was completing the task. With the archaic workflows of my EMR, my attention is drawn away from the clinical scenario to the not-so-smart computer in the room.

What was supposed to make the practice of medicine safer and more efficient is, to date, only a gleam in the eye of software designers, politicians and clinic administrators. For those of us in the trenches, it is at least some of the time just a bunch of extra work with very uncertain benefits.

66) A COBBLER'S MISTAKE

I saw Billy G. yesterday afternoon on his way home from work. He was thrilled to be back to work again. A cobbler's mistake cost Billy two weeks' pay, and it could have cost him his foot.

Billy has had diabetes since he was a teenager, and he has such severe diabetic neuropathy (nerve damage) that he has no feeling at all in his feet. He needs special diabetic shoes, which his insurance company will only replace every several years. They will help him pay to have his work boots re-soled, however, and this got done a month or so ago. Our local cobbler did the job for him while he waited. Billy didn't notice that a week after he got the boots back, the nails used to attach the new soles started to work their way through the sole of his left work boot and the sole of his left foot.

Billy's wife, Theresa, checks his feet for him every night because he isn't quite limber enough to see the bottoms of his feet; some people use a mirror in order to see their feet better, but Billy's diabetes has affected his eyesight too much for him to do the job himself. If Theresa hadn't spotted the wound the first day, who knows what could have happened to Billy's foot. It took two weeks to heal the damage, two weeks without a paycheck, and two weeks of worrying.

Billy went back to the cobbler and told him what happened. Theresa had told me "I suppose we could have sued him, but we just wanted him to know so nobody else got hurt like Billy".

Theresa does one more thing for Billy every day now: Every morning, she checks the inside of his work boots for nails before he puts them on. Then, as she has had to since he started to lose the feeling in his fingertips, she ties his boots for him, and she makes sure they're not tied too tight.

Billy can't feel pain in his feet, but I know he can feel the love in the countless little things Theresa does so that the two of them can carry on day after day.

67) SICKLE CELL DISEASE, LIKE PHENYLKETONURIA IS A GENETIC DISEASE MANAGEABLE WITH DIET

Sickle cell trait is much more common among Africans in Africa than among African-Americans. But sickle cell anemia is more common here. How can that be?

The answer is very simple - EPIGENETICS, specifically your diet.

Not all people with sickle cell trait from both parents get sickle cell anemia. An environmental link had long been suspected and has been known for almost 90 years. I was unaware of it, having grown up and trained in Sweden and working in Maine, two corners of the world with almost no sickle cell anemia cases.

The reason for this difference is that the typical African diet includes cassava and African yam, foods with significant amounts of thiocyanate. Americans with sickle cell trait don't typically eat these foods, and that's why they develop symptoms more often.

In 1932 potassium thiocyanate (KSCN) was used to resolve sickle cell crisis. My reading suggest that this method never did become standard care, and was hardly mentioned at all until 50 years later, when it still didn't become an accepted strategy. Potassium thiocyanate binds through a process called carbamylation to the site of error on the sickle hemoglobin molecule inside the red blood cell and corrects it. The shape and lifespan of the red blood cell are normalized by this reaction.

A 1986 article that tells the story from 1932 even proposed viewing sickle cell anemia as a thiocyanate deficiency anemia affecting people only if they are homozygous for sickle cell trait, rather than a genetically determined disease.

UptoDate mentions hydroxyurea treatment, which can be very toxic, but makes no mention of dietary modification of sickle cell disease at all.

This is an example of EPIGENETICS, factors that affect how our genes (GENOTYPE) may or may not cause disease or other visible attributes (PHENOTYPE). People who are homozygous for the sickle cell trait and still don't get the disease because they eat cassava have the genotype but not the phenotype, if you will.

But it gets even more interesting. While sickle cells are more resistant to the malaria parasite, and cassava eating normalizes the shape and behavior of the red blood cell, this does not increase susceptibility to malaria. This is because cassava provides phytochemicals that weaken the plasmodium falciparum. This is an example of what has been called Human Plant Parasite Coevolution. This is explained in a talk by anthropologist Fatima Jackson. I highly recommend watching it.

So, as the saying goes, we are what we eat, or more accurately, what we eat determines or influences the environment of our genes and their tendency to manifest (express) their potential OR NOT.

All this came to my attention somewhat randomly, and I found it shocking that this isn't more widely known. This knowledge puts Sickle Cell Disease in the same category as PKU, a genetic disease we routinely screen for and prevent by modifying the diet of patients with the PKU genotype. Having had two patients with this disease, born before routine testing started, I am particularly struck by the fact that this old discovery hasn't become common knowledge 87 years after it was first published.

So there it is, PKU (or sickle cell) genotype causes the disease (phenotype) only if the genes are in a certain environment (epigenetics), for example with regards to diet.

68) INTUITING ALEXITHYMIA

"Tell me about the day you passed out," I asked the middle-aged woman in Room 4 the other morning. "How did you feel?"

"We were up early, my husband and I, because Debbie - that's our daughter - was coming home for Easter break. She's on the dean's list at Swartham College. She wants to be a civil engineer with a double in business administration. She's so talented..."

"Were you feeling okay when you woke up?" I tried to redirect her.

"Well, Gordon looked at me kind of funny and asked if I was feeling all right..."

"Were you?"

"He didn't think I looked well. Pasty, he said my face was... Pasty-looking!" She sighed. "I didn't finish my toast or my bran flakes, and I usually gulp my breakfast before Gordon even gets back in the house with the morning paper."

"Did you feel nauseous?"

"I didn't throw up, if that's what you mean. Gordon asked me the same thing. He felt my forehead and said I was clammy."

"Then, what happened?"

"We got ready to go to the airport to pick Debbie up. On the way, I asked Gordon to stop at Dunkin' Donuts and get me some Munchkins, but he was worried we'd be too late, so he talked me out of it."

I started to be increasingly aware of the time.

"Do you remember the moments before you passed out? What did you feel?" I asked.

"I remember thinking it was hot in the luggage hall, and I remember Debbie talking about her new roommate. Then Gordon said he should have stopped for Munchkins after all, because we had had plenty of time and I was probably getting a low blood sugar..."

I changed my strategy and asked several more directed, yes-or-no questions. I formulated a plan for what kind of workup to do.

The rest of the day I kept thinking about that encounter. Over the years I have seen so many patients who don't seem to be able to describe or even recognize their own feelings, but instead tell me what other people notice about how they appear to them. I have often wondered if there was a name and a psychological profile for people like that. They are a challenge to take a medical history from, but they must also be challenged themselves by never really knowing how or what they feel.

Last night after supper, I googled my question.

"Inability to describe own feelings, relying on other people's description" I typed.

The third link on my search gave me the word I needed: "What is alexithymia?" The literal meaning of a-lexi-thymia is "lack of words (for) emotion". I searched for "alexithymia" and a half-dozen articles completely captured my attention.

What I read resonated with my own observations. Curiously, the first website I looked at had been posted or updated the day before my search and the original article by P.E. Sifneos, introducing the word and describing the phenomenon, was published in 1973 - the year before I started medical school. It took me this long to "discover" it myself!

Alexithymia is not classified as a disease in DSM-IV, the psychiatric book of diagnostic definitions. It is rather more like a personality type. What I found fascinating as I read along is the link between alexithymia and psychosomatic illness.

People with alexithymia can't tell if their bodily sensations represent physical or emotional phenomena, because they have trouble registering their emotions. They are likely to look for physical illness as an explanation for sensations others may easily recognize as related to strong emotions. An extreme example from one of the websites I read was that a crying alexithymic might worry about having a blocked tear duct instead of registering their sadness. A person with little insight into how upset, sad or anxious he or she might be would not have any ability to judge whether they might feel bad, be it headache, chest pain or belly cramps, for emotional reasons.

One article suggested up to 10% of people have some degree of alexithymia.

Those impromptu few minutes on the computer made me a wiser clinician. I will be more tenderhearted with patients who have trouble describing their feelings in a fifteen-minute visit, and I will look harder for that trait in patients whose symptoms baffle me.

69) THE MAN WITH THE SHRINKING LUNG

I see some odd things in my clinic. One recent diagnostic dilemma was a man in his late fifties with shortness of breath.

He had been born with a Ventricular Septal Defect and had undergone surgery for this in his infancy. During his lifetime, he had seldom gone to doctors, and always thought he was in fairly good health, maybe just of a weak constitution. A smoker since age 13, he had a morning cough and got a little winded running up and down the basement stairs or shoveling snow in the winter.

A while ago he came to see me because he felt he was getting more short of breath over the winter. On exam, his vital signs were normal and his oxygen saturation was 97%. He had a systolic heart murmur and his breath sounds were diminished in his entire left lung. I didn't see any swelling of his legs and his neck veins were not distended when he laid down flat on my exam table. His EKG was normal.

I ordered a chest X-ray and some basic blood work. His X-ray report said his left lung looked normal but his mediastinum was shifted a little to the left. His heart was not enlarged. Routine labs were normal.

The day he came in to follow up on his testing he looked ashen. He had suddenly become much more short of breath the day before, just brushing snow off his car. He had had some vague chest pressure that lasted ten or fifteen minutes.

His physical exam and repeat EKG were essentially unchanged; perhaps he had even weaker breath sounds in his left lung. This time his oxygen saturation was only 90%.

I ordered a chest CT with contrast for later the same day and also put in for a chemical stress test and an echocardiogram.

A few hours later, one of the radiologists called me. The man's IV had infiltrated and most of the contrast ended up in the subcutaneous tissues of his right arm. His Pulmonary Embolism protocol CT scan would have to be postponed.

"Ok, have him stop by the office on his way home", I said.

I gave him samples of one of the new anticoagulant medications that just got approved for initial treatment of blood clots in the lung and gave him a lot of detailed instructions.

Over the next two weeks, I received a normal stress test and an echocardiogram report that said something about decreased flow across the pulmonic valve. I wasn't sure what to make of that in the context of my working diagnosis of one or multiple pulmonary emboli, and called radiology to please get the chest CT rescheduled.

Finally, this Monday, he had his CT scan done. The chief if radiology called me immediately after the study.

"Your Mr. Faulkner, he doesn't have a PE, but he has agenesis of his left pulmonary artery."

I sat back in my chair. I'd never heard of this condition. All his life, I thought, his underdeveloped left lung has been without functioning blood supply, and that's why his mediastinum was shifted to the left and his breath sounds were so diminished. Finally, all this caught up with him, and he ended up in my clinic one day.

I did an Internet search for pulmonary artery agenesis. It is extremely rare, and usually diagnosed earlier in life. Some cases are diagnosed after an incidental abnormal routine chest X-ray. Symptoms are shortness of breath and productive cough or recurrent respiratory infections, all common concerns among middle aged smokers in this part of the country during the winter months.

I saw him back to explain what I had found, stopped his blood thinner and told him I wanted him to see a specialist at Cityside Hospital. He wasn't so sure he wanted to travel that far, but said he'd think about it.

As a rural frontline primary care doc, you just never know what's going to walk through your door.

70) THE MAN WITH THE UP AND DOWN BLOOD PRESSURE

Gordon Grass had fallen three times. He said he was always lightheaded.

A slender chain smoker with nicotine-stained fingertips, he didn't go to doctors much. He was on a blood pressure pill, though, started years ago by a colleague over in Danderville.

I looked at his vital sign display in my EMR. His blood pressure had never been high in the years that I had known him. In fact, sometimes it was on the low side. His typical systolic blood pressure was 130-134, but occasionally it was in the 100-110 range.

His exam was unremarkable when I saw him a couple of weeks ago. I listened carefully for bruits in his carotid arteries, did a standard neurological and ENT exam and even took out my tuning fork to check his Weber and Rinne; everything was normal.

Sitting on my stool opposite Gordon in the drafty, north facing Room 4, its old windows rattling as a powerful nor'easter pounded on the brick walls of the former hospital, I pulled the portable blood pressure cuff stand closer and tightened it on Gordon's right arm. Sitting, his blood pressure was 136/68, and standing, it was 122/60.

"I think we should stop your blood pressure pill and see how you do", I said. Gordon said he was happy to get rid of them, and we agreed to check his blood pressure and his symptoms in a couple of weeks.

I knocked on the door to Room 1 and entered the sun-drenched room across the hall from where I had seen him two weeks earlier.

"Feel that solar heat", I said as he squinted in the warm, bright yellow room. "How are you doing?"

"Better, not as lightheaded."

I looked at his vital signs. Autumn had entered his blood pressure when she checked him in: 112/62.

"Your blood pressure is lower than last time", I mumbled, adding "I have read that the effect of hydrochlorothiazide can last for months after you stop it."

Instinctively, and without speaking, I pulled the wall mounted sphygmomanometer down from the concrete wall between Gordon's chair and the exam table on his left, tightened it around his arm and pumped up the cuff. Listening carefully as I released the pressure, I, too, recorded a lower blood pressure than last time: 116/60.

"I like the cuff we used last time better, but let me check your right arm also with this cuff", I said and stretched the tubing across to his right arm. There, his blood pressure was 132/78.

"Hmm, let me check a few things again", I said and ran my fingers along his neck, his collarbones and in his armpits. I put my stethoscope in my ears again and listened to his carotid arteries and his lungs.

Finally, I took both his wrists and found each radial pulse with my index fingers. I took a deep breath and relaxed. Then I sat quietly as my fingertips registered his pulse, bom-boom, first in his right wrist, and, a split second later, in his left.

"This is the first time I've diagnosed this condition in thirty five years", I began.

I explained Subclavian Steal Syndrome to Gordon; how a blocked artery under his left collarbone causes blood to be shunted from the right carotid artery, across the brain, and downward through the left carotid and into his circulation-deprived left arm, stealing some of the blood that was supposed to fuel his brain.

"There are two ways you can get this condition", I said. "One is similar to any blocked artery from smoking and all the other causes of poor circulation, and the other is something constricting the artery from the outside, like a cervical rib or a tumor of the lung".

Gordon made a silent gesture to the pack of Pall Mall cigarettes in his breast pocket.

"Yes, them, either way", I said. "Let me order some tests..."

A few days later, the Chief of Radiology called me: Subclavian Steal, no tumor.

Next week, Gordon meets with a cardiovascular surgeon to discuss a bypass of his blocked subclavian artery, because he is still symptomatic, even without his blood pressure pill.

71) A COUNTRY DOCTOR DUPED

A woman in her mid thirties with a terrible limp and a past surgical history in the dozens became my patient two years ago. Her prosthetic left leg served her well, but her right leg was moving awkwardly because of advanced hip arthritis and a formerly shattered ankle.

She was on long acting morphine and short acting oxycodone. Her Social Security disability insurance didn't cover the long acting form of oxycodone.

She told me several times how much she hated being on narcotics, but they kept her functioning. She was able to do her own housework and she was taking classes in medical coding and billing.

Her pill counts were always correct and her urine drug screens always showed morphine and oxycodone - never anything else.

A year ago, an anonymous caller told Autumn that my patient was injecting her morphine. I saw a couple of scratches on her arms, and she told me she had this nervous habit of picking at her skin. I said that habit could keep her from receiving future prescriptions for pain medications, and I never again saw any marks on her arms or legs.

Last summer, we got an emergency room report from Massachusetts that documented how my patient had presented with symptoms of opiate withdrawal. The story she had told there was that she had lost all her pain medication when her car was broken into at a highway rest area several days earlier. She was dehydrated and needed intravenous fluids.

When I saw her back, she was still shaky, and she asked me not to represcribe her long acting morphine. She said, tearfully, that she was determined to get off her narcotics. Just some oxycodone to take the edge off her pain, but she didn't want to have these drugs in her system all the time, she told me.

Her next drug screen only showed oxycodone and its metabolite, oxymorphone, just as expected.

A few months later, she ended up missing her followup appointment because her mother fell ill and needed emergency surgery. "I stretched my oxycodones", she said, "and I did all right".

"Let me do another drug screen, to prove that you didn't take anything else", I said.

She tensed up, but didn't say anything, except "will the results go up on the new patient portal?"

"As soon as I've signed off on them, yes."

A few days later, the opiate confirmation test came in. Her oxycodone level was medium high, but there was no oxymorphone, suggesting only recent oxycodone intake, but not proving continuous use. That was reasonable as she had been taking her prescription less regularly. But, confusing at first, her morphine level was higher than the assay could measure. There was also a high level of codeine.

I had in front of me a test result that suggested probable heroin use.

I had to check my facts, but needed some extra time to do my research. Meanwhile, she called to inquire about her results. Autumn told her that they probably hadn't come in yet, if they weren't on the portal.

Heroin, also called diacetylmorphine, is rapidly metabolized to 6-monoacetylmorphine (6-MAM), which is six times more potent. Within a few hours, 6-MAM is transformed to morphine and no longer detectable in urine or other body fluids. Street heroin often has some acetylcodeine in it, which is metabolized into codeine.

I checked with the reference lab. They could run a test for 6-MAM, but because it is present only for a few hours, it might still be negative even if my patient was using heroin. The turnaround time for the analysis could be up to a week.

I picked up the phone.

"I've got your opiate confirmation test", I started.

She was silent.

"It shows your oxycodone, but also more morphine than I've ever seen, and some codeine."

She said nothing.

"That is the pattern we see with heroin use. And, in any case, you wouldn't be expected to have that much morphine in your system when you are no longer prescribed morphine, and I never prescribed codeine for you. I have a confirmation test pending for 6-MAM, which is a breakdown product that we see in the body before heroin becomes morphine. But this disappears quickly from the system, so we don't always see it in heroin users", I explained, based on my recent homework.

She still said nothing, except "can you put the result up on the portal so I can look at it?"

That was it. She hung up. I never heard from her again.

A few days later, her 6-MAM report came back. It was positive. I signed off on it, and it went up on the portal.

72) A MOTHERLESS CHILD WITHOUT A FATHER

The young man with chest pains, shortness of breath and heart palpitations had come back for his followup visit.

His thyroid test and blood count were well within the normal range, his EKG was normal and his chest X-ray was declared normal by the radiologist.

We talked some more about his anxiety and poor sleeping habits. We talked about his late shift at work, and we talked about his late gaming habits on the computer and how he sleeps until ten and misses out on mornings with his young daughter. He had been setting his alarm and getting up two hours earlier than he used to. That had made him more tired and less inclined to stay up past one o'clock in the morning.

We talked about how many years it had been since his mother died, and the emptiness he had felt ever since then. We talked about how he has had to mother himself in some ways ever since then.

We talked about how he had now gone from being a motherless child to a young father, and I asked him what kind of father he wanted to be for his little girl.

That's when he said, "I wish my dad would act more like a father".

"Do you wish he would give you some more guidance?" I left it open ended.

"Yeah, I feel insecure, like I'll mess up with the baby."

"Have you asked him?"

"Not in so many words. But, he doesn't seem that interested. He'll take me out to lunch and we eat without saying all that much and here he is, fifty years old, texting his girlfriend like some teenager instead of talking with me. I'm scared, I don't know exactly what I'm supposed to do or be like, and he is no role model at all."

"So if your father acted exactly the way you need him to, what would that look like?" I asked.

He thought for a while, and then, with words that flowed on a river of silent tears, he painted a touching picture of a a young father and a still young grandfather talking about what it takes to be a man.

"See, you have a pretty good idea of the kind of advice you would get, then", I said. "And your wife and daughter, what kind of man do you imagine they wish you will turn into as you mature and continue to evolve? Do you think you know that?"

He nodded.

"I understand that you wish your father could help you more, but for whatever reason, he isn't able to give you what you need right now, but it sounds like you already know what kind of man you want to be like."

He nodded again.

"Be the kind of man you wish he was, be the father you want your little girl to have. She will teach you, just watch her and listen. And talk, really talk, with your wife."

With the image still in my mind of the fifty year old man texting his girlfriend while his son pined for his love and attention, I added:

"Maturity and age don't always move along at the same speed. I think you're growing up faster than many people your age."

He shook my hand, very firmly, and said:

"Thanks, Doc."

73) "HELP ME!"

He seemed like his usual self, strong willed and irreverent, with his gravelly voice and nicotine stained fingers, and as always tied with clear plastic tubing to the oxygen concentrator on the back of his wheelchair.

He is a DNR, Do Not Resuscitate. But during his last hospitalization he ended up intubated and on a ventilator for several days.

His daughter gave her version of what happened and the discharge summary was less clear cut. So I turned to him and asked:

"So what happened? How did you end up on a respirator as a DNR?"

He answered "I said HELP ME, and that's what they did".

"I think the doctors panicked when he said that", his daughter concluded.

"And would you want that to happen if you say HELP ME again?"

"No."

"So when somebody can't breathe, there are sometimes only two options, sticking a tube down their throat and hooking them up to a respirator or giving them morphine to treat the agony and anxiety of the process."

I glanced over at his daughter and then looked him straight in his eyes.

"So, let me make sure I hear you right. If you can't breathe and say HELP ME, does it mean machine or morphine?"

"Morphine", he said, emphatically.

I'm glad we had this talk. This very plain talk.

74) DRUG REHAB, LIFE HAB(ILITATION)

We do two things when we treat young adults with opioid use disorder in our Suboxone clinic.

The obvious one is providing the chemical that attaches to certain opiate receptors and quiets cravings without feeding the reward cycle.

Because buprenorphine is also a Kappa antagonist, it has antidepressant and anxiolytics properties that traditional opioids don't have.

By prescribing Suboxone, we help our patients' brains return, partly or completely, to the way they functioned before they became habituated to opioids.

The other thing we try to do, although it isn't just our job, but that of everyone who cares about a young adult in recovery, is habilitation.

Habilitation isn't relearning what you used to know, but acquiring skills you never had in the first place.

We generally say that your emotional and character development stops when you become addicted. It can also arrest when you suffer trauma. The life lessons of cause and effect, immediate and delayed gratification, giving and taking, joy and sadness, self and community are all skipped over to some degree when you are on a chemical roller coaster or suppressed by the weight of emotional trauma.

In our group therapy, facilitators and participants challenge newcomers who feel the world owes them things they haven't earned. We talk about sticking with a job you don't like to build a resume for better jobs in the future. We talk about proving to the DHHS that you can be appropriate and responsible with your children. We talk about making new social contacts and friendships, developing new interests and about coping with stress, emptiness and disappointment.

We have also started a group for friends and families of people in recovery. This group, aided by veteran Suboxone patients, serves as a sounding board for our journey. Because it isn't a paved highway - the prescription part is pretty straightforward, but the other part is different for every patient, every group and every community. It must be local, a grassroots effort.

A lot of interest and a lot of money is flowing into opiate dependence treatment right now, mostly the chemical part.

But once that happens we must face the next big challenge, which isn't talked about much yet, of helping a large cohort of young adults catch up from a decade or two of skipping classes in the school of life.

75) THE MAN WITH BROWN FINGERNAILS

I had seen him now and then, but he didn't come in very often. He was on the thin side, a hard core smoker with chronic bronchitis. But he was still running some borderline blood sugars, a quick chart review revealed.

One day, he came in with a few months of increased "arthritis" in his shoulders, neck, back, knees and hips. There was no sign of small joint synovitis, but the range of motion in his shoulders was poor, and he had a little trouble getting up from his chair without using his arms.

"Polymyalgia Rheumatica?", I thought, but also remembered how people with lung cancer can develop all kinds of musculoskeletal pain. He had had a screening chest CT not too long ago. So I ordered a sedimentation rate and prescribed some low dose prednisone and asked him to come back in a week.

A week later he was only a little more limber, and his sed rate was only 28, not exactly diagnostic.

As I sat there and looked at him, thinking about what to do next, I made the observation that his skin was a little dark for the time of the year and his ethnic background. Then I looked at his fingernails, brown. Not just the ones that held his cigarette, but all of hem, even his pinkies.

I quickly clicked to his lab section in the EMR to check what kinds of lab tests had been done over the past year or so. His CBCs had not changed much over the past few years, and I had just checked one when I did his sed rate. His chemistry profiles had been okay except for those borderline blood sugars. Nothing more had been checked.

"What?" I thought to myself.

"Hyperpigmentation, Addison? No symptoms, and the nails…"

"Iron", was my next thought. "Could he have hemochromatosis?"

I've never diagnosed a case of it before.

"It is possible that all these pains could have something to do with your iron levels", I told him. "I hate to do this, but would you mind giving us some more blood for some extra testing?"

Sure enough, his iron level was elevated. I made a referral to hematology.

I was away for a little while and my first day back he was in my schedule for "Followup blood sugars". He had seen a colleague for urinary frequency and turned out to have a very high random glucose and a glycosylated hemoglobin of 8. He had fallen into the trap of quenching his thirst, which was caused by spilling sugar in his urine, with juice and soda.

Scanning further in the EMR, I saw that the hematology report was back. It spelled out all the possible complications of hereditary hemochromatosis: Joint pain, fatigue, unexplained weight loss, abnormal bronze or gray skin color, abdominal pain, cirrhosis, diabetes, heart disease…

The lesson for me was the nail discoloration, which isn't often mentioned in the medical texts; I remember noticing it before, but always assumed it was just nicotine staining. I never looked at all his nails. And I should have.

76) A NICE, CLEAN DOUBLE WIDE

Driving back from town this evening, I noticed that Marguerite Brown's old farmhouse was gone. For two years now, Marguerite has been talking about how the old homestead was to be torn down, but there never seemed to be a timeline.

Two years ago, just before winter, Marguerite announced proudly that she wasn't spending another winter in that cold, drafty old farmhouse of hers. I had been there years before and remembered it as untouched pre-world war II. The kitchen floor was made of unfinished narrow pine boards, the wooden cabinets were naturally darkened by age, and the woodstove was the only source of heat in that part of the house. The old furnace blew some hot air into the main portion of the house, but here, too, woodstoves made the temperature more bearable on cold evenings.

After Marguerite's husband passed away, she took in a succession of old men as boarders. They got taken care of, and I'm sure it worked for Marguerite, too. That's how I came to see the inside of her house, doing house calls for the elderly men she took care of. A few years ago, she gave up doing that, and soon after, she started talking about not wanting to spend winters in that house anymore. Like many people around here, she decided to get "a nice, clean doublewide", essentially two mobile homes joined into one after delivery.

She sold the acreage in the way back of her property, had her new doublewide put up behind the old farmhouse, and for a couple of years, she chipped away at going through its contents.

"You can't imagine how much junk you gather in sixty years", she told me. She loved her doublewide, and she often told me how glad she was to be out of her old house, but she seemed to take an awfully long time going through its contents and getting ready for its demolition. I suspected it wasn't just a matter of going through the physical contents of the house, but also saying goodbye to the memories of the place where she spent all of her adult life, raised her children, grew old, nursed her husband through the illness that took his life, cared for a succession of elderly boarders, and then spent years alone.

Three weeks ago her eldest daughter, Molly, succumbed to pancreatic cancer. As I drove past the pile of rubble that was left of Marguerite's house today, I wondered if losing her first born child made her finally tear down the old homestead. One more painful memory associated with it...

When I saw her last, she had asked out loud why her daughter had to die, and not her. Then she had added: "No parent should have to bury a child".

The house where Marguerite Brown lived all her adult life, raised her children and became a widow finally got torn down, but as she looks out the front window of her "nice, clean doublewide" I wonder if she won't continue to see it there, even now that it's gone.

77) A DEADLY INTERACTION

I, like most primary care physicians, have many patients on chronic "blood thinners". Warfarin, essentially the same chemical as rat poison, is the most common drug we use, and it can be difficult to manage. Because its effects are counteracted by vitamin K, simple dietary changes like eating fewer or more greens can change the effects of warfarin. There are also many drug interactions to keep in mind.

Because of these interactions we never assume that patients can stay on the same dose of warfarin indefinitely. Some people's numbers vary enough to warrant testing a few times per week. Our clinic's minimum standard is that even stable patients get a blood test once a month to monitor the medication's effect.

We measure the "prothrombin time", or how many seconds the blood takes to clot, and "INR", International Normalized Ratio, which is, roughly speaking, how long a patient's blood takes to clot compared to an untreated person's blood. We typically strive for an INR of 2 to 3, which is 2 or 3 times the normal, untreated, clotting time.

Antibiotics are among the most common drugs that interact with warfarin. Only a handful of antibiotics are safe in this regard. Penicillins, cephalosporins and nitrofurantoin are choices we don't worry about. Azithromycin sometimes interferes, and common urinary antibiotics like sulfa and ciprofloxacin almost always interfere to some degree.

Florence Fitch, an elderly patient of mine with atrial fibrillation, had a urinary tract infection and had seven days of ciprofloxacin prescribed by another doctor. She ended up in the hospital with an intestinal hemorrhage and needed two units of blood.

Today I saw Gwen Hubert. She has high cholesterol and atrial fibrillation. She must have been on warfarin and simvastatin for ten years. Her numbers were always quite stable. When I saw

Gwen the last time, she had complained of fairly significant muscle aches. Her cholesterol was perfect and her creatine phosphokinase (CPK) test didn't show any sign of muscle damage. Still, even when there is no damage, people on simvastatin as well as all the other statins can have bothersome muscle aches.

At our last visit, Gwen and I agreed that she would not take the simvastatin for three to four weeks. If there was no difference, she was to start her cholesterol pill again and see me a month or so later.

She had had an INR drawn the other day and her level was high enough that we had called her to tell her to skip a day of warfarin and start taking a lower dose after that.

Gwen was concerned when I saw her.

"I've never had a high INR before. Do you think starting the simvastatin again caused a problem with my warfarin?"

I looked at her flowsheet. About the time we stopped her simvastatin her INR had dropped. I hadn't thought much of it and just increased her warfarin dose a little. The following week her number was higher, but still not in range, so we had her increase her dose some more. That took care of it. Then, when she started the simvastatin again, her INR went up to 4.

"I haven't seen simvastatin do that before, but I'll look it up."

Our usual drug interaction website didn't respond. The first result on my Google search was an abstract of an article (http://www.ncbi.nlm.nih.gov/pubmed/17565042) from Oslo, Norway, published in 2007:

"An 82-year-old white female was admitted to the hospital because of an international normalized ratio (INR) value greater than 8, which was detected at a routine follow-up visit to monitor warfarin therapy.

Four weeks earlier her lipid-lowering therapy had been switched from atorvastatin 10 mg daily to simvastatin 10 mg daily. She had been treated with 2.5 mg of warfarin daily for almost 30 years due to episodes of deep venous thrombosis and lung embolism. Her INR had been stable within the treatment range (2.0-3.5) for more than 2 years before the INR increase. Upon hospitalization, she was given 5 mg of vitamin K orally. A few hours later she lost the feeling and movement of her right arm and a computed tomography scan showed major bleeding in the left cerebral hemisphere. She died the following day.

DISCUSSION: One study has shown a lack of interaction between warfarin and atorvastatin. In comparison, 3 studies have shown significant increases (10-30%) in warfarin effect and/or reductions in dose requirement after starting concomitant simvastatin treatment. The interaction mechanism between simvastatin and warfarin is not known but is possibly associated with reduced elimination of warfarin. Use of the Naranjo probability scale showed that the likelihood of warfarin-induced INR increase following the switch to simvastatin was probable.

CONCLUSIONS: Atorvastatin and simvastatin appear to differ in their potential to interact with warfarin. Clinicians should be aware of the interaction risk when starting simvastatin treatment in patients on warfarin therapy."

In Gwen's case, restarting a drug she had been on for over a decade could have had the same deadly effect.

78) NOT ON A SILVER PLATTER

The clues are usually there, even in the hardest of cases. They just aren't presented to you on a silver platter.

Gwen Stephenson had an ill-defined polyarthritis and had been on methotrexate for some time. Her rheumatologist, Norm Fahler, had tapered her off the medication while keeping an eye on her inflammatory markers and they had leveled off at just above the normal range.

Seven or eight years ago, Gwen had suffered a bad bout of sciatica, and a few weeks ago, she had told me her sciatica was bothering her a little again. "Not enough to have those injections yet, mind you", she had said with a grimace and a gesture indicating the length of the needle her pain specialist had used to deposit the steroid in her lumbar epidural space.

The visit when she mentioned her sciatica was a diabetes visit, full of bookkeeping tasks - keeping track of her eye exam, foot exam, microalbumen, blood pressure readings, blood sugar log, lipid management and cardiovascular review of systems.

I accepted her assessment that her sciatica was not of the magnitude that it required any immediate intervention.

After Gwen left, Autumn came into my office to pick up some forms I had signed, and she said:

"Did you notice that Gwen's temperature was 99 for the second time in a row? I wasn't sure if I should have pointed that out to you."

I had not noticed it. Looking back, I saw that a week earlier, when she had come in just for her B-12 shot, it had also been 99.

"I'm not sure if that means anything", I remember saying.

Two days later, Gwen came in with a nasty cough and I thought I could hear some very faint rales in her lower left lung. Her temp was 99.4 and I put her on antibiotics for pneumonia. We didn't have X-ray available that day, but it was obvious at that time she needed an antibiotic.

The following evening I was on call. Gwen phoned the answering service around 9 pm and asked if an axillary temperature of 103 was high enough to be alarming. She hadn't been able to take an oral temperature because her teeth were chattering with the terrible chills she was having.

She was admitted to the hospital, where intravenous antibiotics were started for her apparent pneumonia. Her fever didn't come down, and the radiologist disagreed with the initial emergency room reading of her chest X-ray. So she became a "fever of unknown origin". The blood cultures that were drawn in the emergency room grew staphylococci, and, because her back pain kept getting worse as she lay in bed day after day, she had an MRI of her lumbar spine. This showed a possible discitis at L5-S1 and a psoas abscess.

They teach you in medical school that early imaging isn't indicted with back pain or sciatica, unless there are "red flag symptoms". Fever is one of them. But Gwen's back pain was recurrent, and had been there for a while, and her fever was borderline when I saw her, and it developed after the back pain. Still, I was quite humbled. I wasn't actively connecting all the dots, and I was too focused on the housekeeping tasks of her diabetes care to see the subtle manifestations of her smoldering infection.

79) A VERY CAREFUL DRIVER

"I don't know why Dr Brown took my license away", the 92-year old man said. He was visibly shaking with anger. "I've been driving since I was a young boy, and I could find my way to California without a map".

My associate, Dr. Wilford Brown, had sent in a State Driver Profile a few months ago, and made reference to an attached letter by a family member, which in his words would be "very damning, if true". Apparently, the Department of Motor Vehicles had thought so too, as the elderly man explained their action through clenched jaws.

"I called them up, and they said that if you wrote to them, they would give me my license back".

"They did, huh..." I said, while mousing and clicking my way back and forth in the documents section of the electronic medical record in search of the damning letter. I could not find it.

"How could Dr. Brown say that I'm not a good driver? What does he know about that?" The man raised his trembling hand and pointed in the general direction of Dr. Brown's office.

"He says I have memory problems. My memory is excellent. I remember everything!"

I looked at his problem list, where "Dementia" was the first diagnosis.

"Maybe someone contacted the DMV about your driving", I said cautiously, thinking I wouldn't want to cause conflict or mistrust in the family by revealing everything I knew about the letter. "Maybe someone didn't like the way you drive", I tried, wondering if perhaps the missing letter might have been inaccurate or exaggerated.

I looked at his birth date on the computer screen and did a quick search in my memory bank about old cars.

They were still making Model T Fords when he was a little boy. Maybe he even learned to drive in one. I pictured traffic around here in those days, and my mind suddenly switched to the tourist traffic on Route One every summer weekend.

"My memory is excellent", Mr. Gordon said again.

"Well, it's not just memory, it's eyesight, hearing, reaction time, judgement and reflexes", I started.

"I am a very careful driver", he interrupted. "When I come to an intersection, I stop, even if the light is green, and I look both ways before I go".

As in a movie flashback, I saw him as a young boy, sitting next to his father, honking a rubber and brass horn and proudly maneuvering a Model T on an empty country road, surrounded only by cow pastures and potato fields.

"Well, Mr. Gordon", I began. I knew what I had to do.

80) GOOD, STRONG HEARTBEAT, 140 AND REGULAR

"Welcome back. How was your trip? Or exile... you were away for a long time."

"Almost a year", my nine o'clock patient answered. A woman just over forty, she looked tan and physically strong. Her short hair was peppered with gray, different from the last time I saw her. She had gone abroad on assignment for a magazine and a film production company, and before she left, she had joked that she would have to be her own doctor until she could come back to see me again.

"So, what's going on", I asked.

"I'm pregnant, pretty far along. I thought it was early menopause, like my mother and my sister, but that doesn't come with morning sickness. And I can feel my uterus."

"And you haven't seen a doctor?"

While getting ready on my exam table, she told me about her work in small villages far away from clinics or hospitals and her decision not to seek care until she came back home.

Her uterus almost reached her navel. I took out the hand held vascular Doppler we use to measure blood pressures at the calf of people with circulation problems. I changed the probe to the one used for fetal heart tones, an attachment I had never used in my clinic; I stopped doing obstetrics the day I graduated from my residency thirty years ago.

"I never thought I would be pregnant again after my miscarriage when I was twenty-five", she said with sadness in her voice as I applied gel to her abdomen and turned on the device.

There was the loud, swoshing sound of the placenta following her own elevated pulse rate. I pressed deeper and aimed the instrument downward with all kinds of static from the movement against her skin. Then, suddenly, there it was, rapid and perfectly regular; a sound I hadn't heard for thirty years.

"Is that the baby?"

"Sure is." I counted. "Good, strong heartbeat, 140 and regular".

She reached down and grabbed my hand.

"Please leave it there. I want to listen to it longer."

Her eyes moistened and her lips began to quiver. She placed her top teeth on her lower lip as if to keep it still. I rested the probe and we both listened in silence.

I remembered that sound, the rapid heartbeat of unborn babies, from many long nights on duty during the sleep deprived years of residency. I remembered catching a few moments' rest in the on-call room down the hall from two or three monitors with intertwining rhythms of babies waiting to be delivered.

Vividly, I remembered my first delivery, a precipitous double footling breech with no other doctor on the ward than this frightened first-year resident. Just in time, as I stood there with my right hand assessing the situation, old Doc Walker appeared in his street clothes in the delivery room door.

"What'ya got, son? Nurses tell me you got two feet there."

"Yessir," I tried not to quiver.

Doc Walker's slow and gentle words calmed the young mother and guided my hands as they in turn guided the baby, feet first, across the symphysis and onto his mother's belly.

As the Doppler continued to tap out its rhythm, I remembered faces with smiles and tears, happy couples and frightened, single young mothers in the delivery rooms. I remembered blue babies, me slipping in umbilical catheters, the neonatal intensivists watching and supervising.

I remembered my own son, hooked up to an apnea monitor at my own hospital. Years later, as a new grandparent, I was a visitor, strangely out of place in a different neonatal intensive care unit, watching my granddaughter through the walls of an incubator.

Thirty years since I heard that kind of heart sound, and it still touched me in inexplicable ways. I remembered, my whole body remembered, the mixed feeling of dread and excitement when my pager used to go off in the middle of the night: "Call 2350 STAT."

Thirty years ago, I saw more births than deaths. Now I only attend departures. For a minute or two that morning I was again participating, ever so briefly, in the greatest miracle a physician is privileged to be part of.

81) THE ELFINS RETURN

I have known him for over thirty years. He has been legally blind for the past five. He tends to be a practical, no nonsense man. The other day, he seemed restless and very concerned as he lowered his voice and said:

"I don't want you to come to the conclusion that I'm crazy, but I'm seeing things..." he began, "I'm seeing children with elfin faces..."

His large, thin hands were in his lap. I put mine on his and said "I know what that is. You're not crazy. This is something that often happens to people with very poor eyesight. It's called Charles Bonnet Syndrome, and it was actually described in 1760 by a Swiss philosopher who observed it in his grandfather who was going blind. It's like the brain fills in the empty spaces, and for reasons we don't understand, much of the time it tends to be with elfin like children. They're usually friendly and jovial and there's nothing threatening about them."

"Right, these are. I'm so glad to hear this is not some psychosis."

"It's a hallucination, but not a psychosis", I reassured him. I printed up an article and gave it to him to show his friends and the staff at the Senior Citizens Home.

A few days later I heard how appreciated the article was.

This was only the second time in my career I have seen this condition. The first time I had no idea what it was but a family member of that patient brought in a printout of an article they had googled. That was ten years ago and I wrote about it in my first year of blogging. Apparently up to 10% of people with visual acuity under 20/60 have this syndrome, and it tends to go away when vision is completely lost.

This little incident evoked two distinct feelings for me. The first one was the comfort, confidence and gratitude that I could instantly reassure my longtime patient that what he was experiencing has happened to other people and has a name and a long history. The other feeling was equally profound and mixed with all kinds of emotions:

My patient was once my neighbor, and my soon to be 35 year old son was often hanging around his yard, checking out his motorcycle, convertible Mustang and garden tractor. My son did look like a little elfin at that time. Maybe it was him that he was "seeing".

82) INSTANT RELIEF

Few things in primary care give patient and doctor mutual and instant gratification.

It's been a while since I reduced a "nursemaids elbow" or a spontaneous shoulder dislocation other than my own, or a finger dislocation, but those all count.

I once wrote about curing deafness in a man with a movement disorder by flushing ear wax more or less on the run as he bobbed around the exam room. That was instantly rewarding and also both exhausting and exciting. Even more ordinary cases of cerumen impaction are rewarding to treat. I almost never let my medical assistants get the satisfaction, or the risk, associated with that procedure.

A few months ago a man came to my Saturday clinic with a plastic tip from his hearing aid lodged sideways deep inside his ear canal. With the help of my modern headlamp (I trained on the cartoonish forehead mirror ENT doctors used to sport) and a delicate long pair of forceps I was able to remove it and relieve the stranger's suffering.

Often, I delight in asking a patient to make the shoulder movements that hurt them so much a few minutes earlier and now feeling no pain, confirming that my steroid-Xylocaine (Hurrah Sweden!) injection hit the right spot.

A few weeks ago I saw a patient for an unrelated problem, who had recently received a nerve block by a nurse practitioner to the minor occipital nerve. The patient had presented with severe pain on the side of her head and the shot gave instant relief. I had never heard of that injection, so I read up on it.

Wouldn't you know it, the following week I saw a different woman with an excruciating pain on the left side of her head. The pain seemed to originate in the back of her head. She was tender on the scalp over her ear and even more so over the lesser occipital nerve. She agreed to an injection. It was instantly successful.

In medical school it was "see one, do one, teach one". This time it was "read about it, then do it". Now I'm ready to teach it, thanks to a clinician with fewer years of education, born well after I started medical school. I'll happily learn from anyone who knows something I don't.

83) A SORE THUMB

It started with a sore thumb and ended with a lifetime of medication. In between there was an emergency room visit at one small hospital, an ambulance transfer to a big hospital, a Medevac flight to Massachusetts General Hospital, multiple invasive procedures and a diagnosis of an often lethal condition. And I was not the one who made that diagnosis.

Paul Allard had developed severe heartburn and indigestion earlier this fall, and had just recovered from a bout of wrist pain when I saw him a month ago. The pain and swelling had been there for a week or so, did not seem to be caused by any trauma or overexertion. It had cleared up after just three days of prednisone, and his rheumatology blood profile was completely negative.

This time, Paul had a pain along half of his left thumb and in the web space between his thumb and his index finger. It was sharp, burning and persistent.

As I asked all kinds of questions and checked his hand strength, skin temperature, monofilament and temperature sensation, arm strength, neck movements, axillary and supraclavicular lymph nodes, Paul clearly seemed uncomfortable. His partner, who usually seemed a little disinterested in Paul's medical concerns, was leaning forward in his chair watching our exchange and my exam intently.

"I'm not sure what's going on", I said to the two men. "It could be something arthritic, like that episode of wrist pain, or maybe some type of vascular inflammation in a very small vein or even one of the four arteries that supply the thumb, but it could also be a pinched nerve, especially because it involves the space between the thumb and index finger."

I suggested that Paul finish the course of prednisone he had been able to stop early when his wrist pain resolved. Paul and John agreed and we set up a five day followup.

That was Friday. Monday morning, my inbox had the next several installments of the story:

Late Friday night Paul suddenly developed nausea, severe abdominal and left flank pain, and went to our small hospital emergency room. They did a CT scan of his abdomen, which showed an infarction of his left kidney. When that happens, the cause is usually a blood clot, so they transferred him to Cityside Hospital for evaluation by the vascular surgeons.

A CT angiogram showed a large clot in Paul's thoracic aorta. He was started on a heparin drip and airlifted to Boston. There, they didn't see the clot in the thoracic aorta, but it had apparently just moved down to his abdomen. The clot was removed surgically, and while his kidney showed signs of recovery, and several specialists were working out his diagnosis, his left lung suddenly filled with blood. He had three quarts of blood drained through two chest tubes and was finally allowed to return to Maine with a diagnosis that explained what had happened and committed him to a lifetime of warfarin to prevent future blood clots.

"So, you have Lupus Antigen", I said, rhetorically. "But they didn't think that you have lupus?"

"Right", Paul and John answered in unison.

"Sure, the wrist pain could have been something else. What did they think of the thumb pain, a small embolus in one of the four little arteries that supply the thumb?"

"They weren't sure", Paul answered.

"Who would have known...", was all I could say.

"He could have died, they told us", John said.

"Most people with this kind of clot do", Paul filled in.

I half shook, half nodded my head as I punched in Paul's warfarin dosing order in the computer. I thought, not for the first time, about how you see things on the front lines of medicine that turn out to be the first sign of a condition that other colleagues diagnose hours, days, weeks or even years later, as symptoms evolve and the clinical picture comes into clearer focus. It is a humbling experience.

It has been said about the Lupus Antibody Syndrome's sister condition, "If you know lupus, you know medicine".

84) ONE MORE QUESTION

"Any recent antibiotics? Steroids?" I asked my last patient of the day, a healthy looking young woman with what she described as a yeast infection that was driving her crazy. She'd had many of them, and they were always coming back, but she had only used over the counter topicals. I knew she needed oral medication, but I asked one more question:

"Any trouble with high blood sugars?"

Her answer eliminated any late day drowsiness or fatigue I might have harbored.

"No, my sugars have always been fine, even during my pregnancies, but I always have sugar in my urine."

"That's why you get all these yeast infections. Has anyone ever looked into why you have sugar in your urine?"

"No."

We got a fingerstick blood sugar, which was low normal, and a urinalysis which showed 4+ glucose, no protein, a pH of 5 and normal specific gravity.

I took a deep breath.

"When the blood is filtered in the kidney, a lot of valuable stuff ends up in the urine, but then we reabsorb things like sugar, because the body is thrifty. You have a kidney disease that keeps you from reabsorbing the sugar. I'm not smart enough to know exactly which variety of disease you have but I'd like to get some more labs tomorrow and refer you to a nephrologist."

She asked for some information about the kinds of kidney disease she might have and added, "well, you're smart enough to know what my basic problem is. I've had it all my life and nobody has said anything about any of this, they were just happy that my blood sugar was okay."

A seemingly ordinary symptom, one additional piece of history and distant memories from medical school, never touched since then...

How can you not be fascinated by this job?

85) JUMPING TO CONCLUSIONS

Muffy Wahl slipped backwards on her icy porch and landed on her right hip. Bruised and sore, she took it easy for a few days but she still went to her exercise class the following Thursday. The petite sixty-three year old was determined not to let a silly little fall set her back, and she did her jumping jacks to the loud, fast music with more determination than usual. She could barely drive herself home afterwards.

After dinner Thursday night she didn't know what to do with herself; she shifted her weight back and forth, but the pain was just as bad no matter how she positioned herself. Getting ready for bed she noticed the bruises were bigger and now reached around to her groin.

Even flat on her back she was in pain. It was a constant, relentless, nauseating pain unlike anything she had experienced before.

Friday morning she got a call from her twin sister, Mary, who had just been admitted to the hospital with a hip fracture. Muffy promised to go and see her, even though it meant a twenty-mile drive. She took some ibuprofen and drove off to see her sister.

After the two women had visited for a while, Mary noticed Muffy's pained expression as she shifted her weight in her chair. Mary suggested that Muffy get herself checked out downstairs in the emergency room. Muffy hesitated, still thinking it was just a bad bruise. Besides, she had never had any dealings with St Bartholomew's Hospital; she always went to Cityside.

Mary insisted, and soon Muffy was downstairs, wearing a hospital gown and being wheeled into x-ray.

"The x-rays were normal and they said it was just a bad bruise", Muffy told me Monday afternoon in the office "Then they gave me a shot for pain that wouldn't make me tired. I drove myself home later on."

"And then..." I asked.

"I noticed the welts Saturday morning. I've been in agony all weekend."

"Welts?"

"Yes, I thought it might have been an allergic reaction to the shot they gave me, but they were only around my right hip."

"Let me see", I said.

She exposed the skin around her right hip. There were bruises, red blotches, and the unmistakable blisters of Herpes Zoster - shingles.

"This is shingles. Did anyone look at your skin?" I asked.

"No, they checked how my hip moved and took the x-rays through the hospital gown", she answered.

86) "WHEN I WAS YOUR AGE"

"Listen, when I was your age, I did the same thing..."

The words came out of my mouth too fast for my frontal cortex to weigh them or to monitor, let alone modulate, the intensity of my delivery.

He was a relatively new patient, 17 years old, scheduled for a well child exam. A tall, athletic young man, he was alone in the exam room. His right arm was in a sling.

"What happened to you?" I asked.

He started telling me about how his right arm got pulled out of its socket a week earlier and how the emergency room had done an X-ray and a CT-scan that were both negative.

There was a knock on the door and Autumn produced the ER note and the radiology reports. The disposition was to see the on-call orthopedist at Cityside within a few days.

"Did you get an appointment with the orthopedic doctor? It says here you were supposed to see him within a couple of days", I said.

He shook his head, adding "but it doesn't hurt as much as it did the first couple of days. My dad told me to climb the wall with my fingers like this.."

"I wouldn't do that until the orthopedist says it's okay", I interjected. "Let me call Dr Fazad and see what's going on with your appointment."

I pulled my old Motorola from my pocket and called. My young patient looked at the clock on the wall. Dr. Fazad's office said they didn't have anything from the ER. "But, he's under 18 so he needs to be seen by pediatric orthopedics", the secretary said. "I'll connect you."

A minute or two later the pediatric orthopedic clinic wanted to know his name and date of birth.

"No, we don't have anything on him, but I can see from the ER note that he needs to be seen. We'll call them later today with an appointment."

I repeated what they had told me and what I had blurted out before.

"Don't do any range of motion exercises until the orthopedic doctor tells you to. Usually you need to be in a sling for six weeks with this type of injury."

His whole body revolted and he got up from his chair.

"Six weeks?!"

"Yes, that's how long it takes for the tissues around the joint to heal. When I was your age I had the same injury. I was away from home and figured since it popped back in, I must be okay. That's why I've dislocated it twenty more times since then."

He cringed at what I said.

"You might even want to tie the sling behind your back", I added.

He gestured toward the loops on his sling that were just for that purpose.

"I say what I say because I wouldn't want you to have to be guarding that shoulder for the rest of your life", I said.

I know you usually can't tell a young person very much - I should have remembered from raising my own children. But I wanted to spare him the complications I suffered from ignoring my injury.

I didn't tell him about the other medical regrets in my life.

A few years after my shoulder dislocation, my grandfather developed double-sided groin hernias, and I didn't know then that two simultaneous hernias sometimes means there is a growing tumor inside the abdomen.

When I was already a young doctor, I watched my mother during one July visit stop and catch her breath now and then in the summer heat. I thought she was just suffering from the heat, and didn't consider paroxysmal atrial fibrillation. She had to have a stroke before that diagnosis was made.

I hope he follows my advice.

87) A TIGHT SQUEEZE

Laura Schwartz could have hour-long spells of squeezing chest pressure, but she was pretty sure it wasn't her heart. After all, she was trim, athletic and by her own admission also a "health nut".

A few years ago she had a stress test with with an abnormal EKG response to exercise but normal nuclear images. The cardiologist we consulted, as most in the cardiac community, felt the normal imaging trumped the abnormal EKG and declared her pain non-cardiac.

Her episodes of chest pressure recurred now and then. We had talked about the possibility of coronary spasm, but she wasn't sure I was right about that. I had seen women before with "Cardiac Syndrome X", who had classic exercise induced angina but normal coronary arteries. They tend to have only a mildly increased risk of actually having heart attacks, and sometimes get better over time on their own. In Laura's case, the chest pain occurred sometimes with exertion like classic angina and sometimes randomly at rest the way Prinzmetal's, or vasospastic angina usually behaves. She seemed to stand somewhere between the different types of angina, or perhaps she had esophageal spasm.

Laura wanted to leave things alone, and kept up her busy life, attending committees, exercising, gardening and maintaining her big house.

But six months ago, the intensity of Laura's chest pressure seemed to intensify, and she was on the verge of accepting a referral for another cardiac consultation. Then she cancelled a couple of appointments and disappeared off my radar screen.

Last month Laura came back with a history of three days of on-and-off squeezing chest pressure. Her EKG was normal, but this time she was as concerned as I was. She accepted an ambulance transfer to the hospital where her first troponin blood test was normal, but the second one was dramatically elevated.

She was transferred from our community hospital to Capital Cardiac Center and underwent urgent catheterization. Bob Googan, one of their senior cardiologists, called me from the cath lab. "Hey, this patient of yours, Laura Schwartz, has normal coronaries but she has apical akinesia and must have infarcted because of spasm, so we'll discharge her on something for spasm.

When I saw Laura in follow-up, she looked and felt great. We talked about how misunderstood women's heart disease still is, and she sighed and said, "I know I have to pace myself. I'm not forty anymore, and I was pushing too hard". She accepted a referral for cardiac rehab.

I am waiting to see if her calcium channel blocker will help prevent her angina, as with typical coronary spasm, or if she will need to be switched to a beta blocker, as many women with Cardiac Syndrome X.

This is the art of medicine.

88) A JUDGMENT CALL

"My name is DeWitt. I'm a neurosurgeon in Charleston, South Carolina," a velvety male voice announced. I cocked the telephone receiver under my chin as I grabbed the chart Autumn handed to me.

"I have just operated on your patient, George Magnusson. He had a large subdural hematoma from a fall that happened a few days ago." The surgeon spoke in a slow, subtle Southern accent. He continued:

"The reason I am calling is that you've had this man on blood thinners for several years now for a pulmonary embolus and deep vein thrombosis he suffered after a motor vehicle accident."

I glanced at Mr. Magnusson's problem list.

"Yes, in 2001," I replied.

"Right," he continued, "but he has a Greenfield filter, so he is protected from pulmonary embolization." After a slight pause he continued in a restrained, low voice:

"I don't believe one usually continues the warfarin under those circumstances. I had to reverse it for the surgery and will be leaving him off it while he's here, obviously. But I would suggest you discuss the risks and benefits with him when he returns home."

"What was his prothrombin time?" I asked.

"It was therapeutic. And I expect him to make a full recovery, fortunately for all of us," he added. "He should be back in your area next week."

The telephone conversation left me thinking.

George Magnusson had taken his blood thinner faithfully for ten years and had hardly ever been out of the therapeutic range. He was fairly healthy otherwise, and I seldom saw him during the three or four years he had been my patient. When I first met him, I had not questioned his need for chronic anticoagulation.

One school of thought is that patients with a definite trigger for a blood clot, such as a major fracture, can be taken off blood thinners after three to six months. Another viewpoint is that patients with a history of massive clots are better left on their blood thinners indefinitely.

Had I failed George Magnusson by keeping him on warfarin and subjecting him to an unnecessary risk of bleeding as he was getting older? After all, his clots happened after a major car accident with multiple fractures.

In my mind I went over what I remembered about inferior vena cava filters. I had very little experience with them, but never thought of them as a replacement for anticoagulation. At best they only reduce the risk that a blood clot would separate from its location in a leg and travel to the lungs, but a person who is at risk for blood clots in the legs could still develop them.

My most trusted online database stated: "Because patients with IVC filters are at risk for IVC thrombosis, insertion site thrombosis, and recurrence of the initial thromboembolic event, continued use of anticoagulants when there are no contraindications is prudent."

When George and Ellen Magnusson returned from their winter vacation near Hilton Head, South Carolina, they both looked tired. George's thick, gray hair had been shaved on one side of his head for the operation.

I went over the pros and cons of staying on blood thinners after trauma-related clots like George's. Especially Ellen looked reserved.

215

"Dr. DeWitt was very sure blood thinners weren't necessary," she said.

"It's a judgment call," I answered. "Why don't we get a hematology consultation? I'd like to hear what someone like Dr. Hertzog thinks about your situation."

Ellen and George left the office and we agreed to talk again after the hematology consultation.

This morning I got a call from the Emergency Room. George just came in with a massive clot from his calf all the way up to his groin.

I guess we won't need that hematology consult, after all.

89) USELESS MEDICINE

Cora Mills had never been treated for asthma before, but when I saw her this winter with a sinus infection and a tight sounding cough, she was wheezing terribly. Her oxygen saturation was fine but her peak flow was in the low normal range. She refused the steroid pills I wanted her to take along with her antibiotic, so I offered her a prescription for an albuterol inhaler.

Cora had never used an inhaler before, so after I wrote her prescriptions, I left her room and got a demonstrator inhaler to show her the proper technique and let her practice a few times.

She had a little trouble coordinating her breathing and activation of the inhaler, so when there was a knock on the exam room door and Autumn, my nurse, announced that the Emergency Room was on the phone, I left Cora to practice on her own a few more times.

The call took longer than I expected, and by the time I got back to Cora's exam room, she was already wearing her long wool coat, felt hat and scarf, ready to leave.

I quickly wrapped up the visit and told her to come back if her chest symptoms didn't clear promptly.

Two months went by, and last week Cora came back in for her annual checkup.

"How'd you make out with your asthmatic bronchitis?" I asked.

"I had a terrible time clearing it up," she quipped. That sample inhaler you gave me didn't do a darn thing for my breathing!"

No wonder I haven't seen my demonstrator inhaler lately, I thought to myself.

"That was a practice device with no medication in it, I explained. I wrote a prescription for the real thing. Do you still have the placebo inhaler we used to practice with?" I asked.

"No, I was so upset with it that I threw it away!" She grinned and shrugged.

90) A LESSON LEARNED

It was late afternoon. The woman who had seen my colleague, Dr. Wilford Brown, a few days earlier was sitting in my exam room. Her chart note read like a typical unnameable virus: Headache, bodyaches, fatigue, low grade fever. She had always seemed like a level-headed resolute woman, but she had called three days in a row for medical advice because she felt so poorly. And it all sounded like a simple virus that a few more days of rest would take care of.

She did have a good sized boil in the middle of her back, but that wouldn't make her feel that sick. The rest of her exam was perfectly normal.

"Let's check your blood count to see if this looks viral", I suggested.

"Anything", she answered.

I moved on to the next patient. A few minutes later I was handed a printout of her CBC. Her white blood cell count was 1.88, almost critically low and without the "right shift" that often accompanies a low WBC in certain viral illnesses. Her platelet count was 68, not far above where spontaneous bleeding might occur.

"I need to send you to the hospital for more testing. I don't know what's going on. It could still be a virus, but you need to be checked for blood poisoning", I explained.

She felt well enough to drive herself to Cityside. For a split second I agonized about that decision. If she was going septic, could she suddenly drop her blood pressure on the way? But I agreed to have her drive.

I called the ER and spoke with one of their regulars about her case.

"Ok, we'll be looking for her", the seasoned but still young physician answered after my thumbnail description of her.

Fifteen minutes later I got another printout. Her ALP, ALT and AST were all about three times the upper normal limit. What wold cause that kind of liver irritation, I thought to myself.

"Fax it to Cityside ER", I told Autumn, and I called back and left a message for Dr. Waterman about the new information.

I told Dr. Kim about her and, without hesitation, he said "I'll bet she has anaplasmosis".

I've seen plenty of Lyme Disease. I grew up with ticks in the country where Erythema Chronicum Migrans was first described. But I hadn't had any experience with anaplasmosis, another tick borne disease, also treatable with doxycycline. I had thought of that as a near tropical disease.

I checked UptoDate and a few other sources, and certainly all the symptoms matched, as well as the low white count and platelets and the elevated liver enzymes. A rash can occur but not usually. The description "summer flu" stuck in my mind from my brief reading.

The next morning I got the admission history and physical. The hospitalists at Cityside suspected a tick borne illness but worked my patient up for sepsis to be safe.

Two hours later, Monica, our new nurse practitioner, asked me to look at a rash. The patient was a woman in her late sixties. The rash consisted of several blanching maculae, each measuring 4-5 inches. None of them were itchy. She was feeling fairly well, but when I asked her about recent illnesses, she said she had been to the ER at Mountain View Hospital the week before with a headache, fever and body aches.

Monica got called away for a telephone call. I sat down by the computer and pulled up the woman's ER report. The labs they had done showed a low white count, a low platelet count and liver enzymes twice the normal limit. I printed up the report.

"I know what this is", I said to Monica when she came back, and handed her the ER note. "It looks like a tick borne illness, possibly anaplasmosis. Why don't you get a tick panel and put her on doxycycline."

(Thanks, Dr. Kim.)

91) PAIN AND SUFFERING

"Suffering ceases to be suffering in some way at the moment it finds a meaning"   Viktor Frankl

"It is much more important to know what sort of a patient has a disease than what sort of a disease a patient has"   William Osler

Back in the 1990's when pain was the newest vital sign, physicians were mandated to treat it, often with powerful medications and without truly understanding the cause and significance of the pain for individual patients.

Plato and Aristotle didn't include pain as one of the senses, but described it as an emotion. The word "pain" is derived from Poine or Poena, the Greek goddess of revenge and the Roman spirit of punishment. Her name is also the origin of the word penalty.

Of course, pain was never measured objectively in antiquity or when it became a "vital sign" a couple of decades ago. It still can't be measured, which makes it no more of an objective clinical sign than someone guessing their temperature without a thermometer.

"Pain and Suffering" is a legal constellation that equates the significance of the two afflictions; doctors, however, have wanted to think of the two as separate, one or the other, treated differently. In many instances, doctors treated only one - the one we call pain - and skirted around the other. We have pain specialists, but perhaps only end-of-life care formally addresses suffering; it is seldom a topic in everyday medicine.

How many times, when a patient has said "I hurt" have I asked "where" instead of "how" or "tell me more", assuming the Chief Complaint is physical.

How many patients with chronic pain are unrelieved by our usual pain medications? And how many of them receive the label "psychosomatic", but little help from their doctors?

A few weeks ago, I came across a short piece by Dr. Thomas H. Lee in The New England Journal of Medicine about suffering. He begins:

"Physicians and health care organizations know that pain, anxiety, uncertainty, and confusion are common among patients, and we work hard to reduce these problems. So why do we avoid the word "suffering," which captures so completely what patients endure?"

I have continued to think about his words ever since.

I think medicine embraced pain assessment and pain treatment in a way that overcompensated for our ineptitude at mitigating suffering. Even as we treat patients' pain, we sometimes cause suffering through the dehumanizing way our clinics and hospitals work.

Dr. Eric Cassell describes suffering as something that happens when our personhood is threatened. Sometimes physical pain, disability or the threat of dying is the cause of suffering, but sometimes the threat to personhood is loss in other spheres. In order to alleviate suffering, physicians need to understand something about the nature and meaning of this threat.

Doctors in our era are trained to treat diseases. We are not often formally trained to explore the person with the disease; this is something we are left to discover on our own, when the disease paradigm doesn't seem to fit the patient we are trying to help.

The movement we now call "narrative medicine" is focused on the subjective meaning of disease and suffering. It offers a way out of the mechanized mindset of evidence-based medicine that is built solely around the lowest common denominators of diagnoses and treatments. The corporate-scientific medicine of today dismisses the statistical "outliers" and individual variations between patients in its efforts to help the greatest number of individuals, instead of each particular patient in the physician's exam room.

Doctoring is a personal calling, built on personal relationships. Even statistical outliers deserve health care that works for them, and suffering can never be understood or mitigated without first seeking knowledge of the suffering person's own fears and beliefs.

Eric Cassell writes:

"The doctor-patient relationship is the vehicle through which the relief of suffering is achieved. One cannot avoid 'becoming involved' with the patient and at the same time effectively deal with suffering."

How many doctors are comfortable getting that involved? And how many health care organizations see that as the role of their physicians?

92) DIAGNOSES RIGHT UNDER MY NOSE

When I read a case report in a journal or whenever a patient comes in to see me about a new symptom, all my senses are tuned in and I know there is a diagnosis to be made.

But on regular clinic days with "routine" follow ups, I find myself not being as tuned in as I would like to be. I know my patients well; we are all growing older together. They change gradually over the years, just as I do. A couple of times last year I have found myself surprised and ashamed that someone else made a new diagnosis in a patient I was seeing on a regular basis.

Stella Sanders world had shrunk since her boisterous husband died a couple of years ago. She had never learned to drive, so without Roy to take her places, she had become virtually housebound. Her spinal stenosis had gone from moderate to severe, and she couldn't take care of her home in the way she had always prided herself in. She admitted she was depressed, but didn't want to take an antidepressant and wouldn't hear of seeing a counselor. Her whole demeanor had changed. She never smiled, and she was less animated in all her facial expressions and body movements.

It was her neurosurgeon who saw it. He had nothing to offer for her spinal stenosis, but he suggested she talk to me about the possibility of her having Parkinson's Disease.

I saw her again the other day, and on Sinemet she looks almost like her old self again.

Fred Nystrom's health had been declining for years, and after going through both an operation for a fractured hip and emergency bowel surgery for perforated diverticulitis last year, he never recovered his old level of functioning. He came back from rehab the second time using a walker. Two months later he was still using it. His affect was flat and he couldn't keep track of his medications the way he had a year earlier. His enlarged prostate seemed to bother him more and more, and he moved too slowly to always make it to the bathroom.

It was my partner, Dr. Wilford Brown, who made the observation that Fred had dementia, gait disturbance and urinary incontinence - the classic triad of normal pressure hydrocephalus. Fred is going in to have a shunt placed to drain his ventricles at the end of this month.

Our challenge is, in the hustle and bustle of everyday practice, to look beyond the issue at hand often enough to "see the big picture" in each patient, and at the same time keep a constant vigil for small changes that could mean a new disease is evolving.

93) A G.O.M.O.

In Emergency Room vernacular, a G.O.M.E.R. is someone whose frequent visits are unwelcome, often an elderly and noncommunicative patients who is sent or dropped off with vague complaints not easily remedied in the ER. The acronym stands for "Get Out of My ER", and it comes from Samuel Shem's novel "House of God".

In my line of work, we have what I think of as G.O.M.O. patients. I don't know if anybody else uses the term, but in my mind it means "Get Out of My Office", specifically "and to the ER instead".

The other day I was called to the lab to see an elderly looking man, who turned out to be my own age (that gave me pause, and maybe I need to do some introspection here...), who looked a little peaked as two phlebotomists were trying to coax him into the phlebotomy chair and off his feet.

"He feels lightheaded", I was told.

"Are you fasting this morning?" I asked.

"Yes", he answered after he landed in the chair.

"Are you a diabetic?" I continued.

"Yes", he said.

"Let's get a finger stick blood sugar", I said. It was 188.

I grabbed a blood pressure cuff. His pulse was 80, and so was his blood pressure. His oxygen saturation was 96%.

"Are you having any chest pain?" I asked.

"No."

"Are you short of breath?"

"A little."

"Did you eat okay yesterday?"

"No."

"Why not?"

"I didn't feel good."

I thought of my blog post "Twenty Questions" as I continued my interrogation.

"In what way did you not feel good?"

Finally, he uttered two dozen words at once:

"I did some yard work yesterday morning and when I came back inside I felt really weak and nauseous so I didn't eat all day."

"Did you have any chest pain then?"

"No."

"Did you have any diarrhea or vomiting?"

"No."

By that time it was clear this man was a G.O.M.O. that needed to go to the ER by ambulance. His EKG was normal, his blood pressure remained low at 80/60 and by the time the EMTs rolled him out of the lab on a stretcher, I had called the ER and we had faxed his medical history to Cityside.

Sometimes all we do is triage, I thought to myself as I sat down at my desk with the M*A*S*H* poster in front of me.

94) AN INNOCENT LOOKING RASH

Ted Hall was in for a blood pressure check and flu shot today. He is a secure, big-boned man with a hint of a southern drawl. A retired military man with a son who is a decorated war hero, he has seen a lot, and seems to take everything in stride.

Wrapping up his visit, I looked at his "Problem list", the cover sheet on the left hand side of the chart that lists his allergies, chronic medical problems, social and family history. A couple of words under "Family History" caught my eye and rekindled my memory. I asked:

"How is Brittany doing?"

He beamed. Brittany was his youngest daughter. I had seen her only once, but I have carried the memory of that June afternoon in my heart for the last 23 years.

It was a stifling hot Thursday afternoon. I was relatively new in town and Brittany Hall was a High School senior, who usually saw a colleague of mine who was off that day. She had a rash on her legs, graduation was the next day, and I agreed to see her as a "double book".

Entering Room 11, the same room where I saw her father today, I met a pretty, blonde girl with a flowery summer dress. She didn't look like most girls from around here, and she carried herself differently. She seemed older and more mature than most eighteen year olds.

Brittany felt fine, and was just concerned about an unsightly bright red rash on both legs. It had been there for a couple of days. She wanted it gone, or at least less noticeable by graduation the next day.

The rash that covered both calves of her fair-skinned legs was petechial and didn't fade when compressed. The rest of her exam was normal.

"These are broken blood vessels," I explained to her. "We need to run some blood tests."

Fifteen minutes later I knew for certain what I had already feared. Her white blood cell count was 28,000, all the same kind of cells - she had acute leukemia, and within twenty more minutes I had arranged for her to meet with the oncologist on call at the hospital twenty miles up the road.

As she left the office with Ted, who came to pick up his daughter, she said:

"And I thought I would just get a cream to put on my legs."

I never saw her again, but the reports from the Cancer Clinic kept trickling in. She went through chemotherapy, delayed long enough so she could attend her graduation, and then she left for college. Ted was my colleague's patient, and I would see him occasionally. Dr. Walls left the area, and Ted became my patient a couple of years ago.

I know I had asked him once before about Brittany, and he had told me she was well, but that time we had not pursued the subject more. Today we lingered more with the story we shared.

"She's 42 now, you know, a beautiful woman" he said, "and she is married and has two gorgeous, healthy children. The cancer doctors had warned her she might never had children, but she had no problems."

"I'll never forget that day she came in with the rash on her legs," I said.

"Me neither," he choked.

95) A QUICK LISTEN

Jack Frommer has been my patient since last fall. He has high blood pressure and high cholesterol and he had a small heart attack six years ago.

Jack hates to take pills, and that was one of our topics when I first met him. He needed some changes in his regimen, based on his history, lab work and physical exam.

We had a lot of ground to cover in that first visit, but I don't remember feeling particularly rushed. Other than his blood pressure, his cardiovascular exam was normal. I re-read my notes the other day. His heart sounded regular without murmurs, his neck veins weren't engorged, his carotid arteries didn't have bruits, and the pulses at his ankles were good and strong. I remember him pointing out as I listened to his neck that nobody had done that before.

His three-month follow-up was encouraging. His cholesterol had dropped below his target level with the new medication I had prescribed, and his blood pressure was almost normal. I spent some extra time on his smoking and the importance of taking aspirin.

I didn't do much of an exam that day because it was a brief visit with a lot of numbers to talk about.

At his six-month follow-up all the numbers looked good. We talked about the 3-4 cigarettes he was still smoking. I listened to his lungs and repeated his cardiovascular exam.

Suddenly, there it was: A loud, harsh scraping bruit in the lower portion of his right carotid artery.

An ultrasound suggested a stenosis greater than 80% and an MRA clinched the deal. Within weeks, Jack had surgery to remove the buildup in his neck artery.

In follow-up he and his wife showered me with praise for saving him from a stroke by listening and noticing the abnormal sound in his carotid artery.

I felt humble. I had not heard it the first time I listened.

96) I'M SORRY MRS. JONES, BUT YOU HAVE ALBUMINUROPHOBIA

Last week I saw several older patients who were fretting about their mildly reduced kidney function. All of them were women in remarkable health, but each one had at one time or another had a brush with hospital medicine:

Mrs. Allard had a mastectomy five years ago, Mrs. Perlman had an episode of clostridium difficile colitis last year after taking antibiotics for a dental infection, and Mrs. Jones had just finished rehab after a knee replacement. All three women had been labeled as suffering from chronic kidney disease during their hospitalization.

Mrs. Allard was in on Monday. She never fails to ask what her Glomerular Filtration Rate is when she comes in for her visits. Every time I have to reassure her that her numbers are stable. She struggles to believe me when I tell her that her frequent urination is not a warning sign of impending kidney failure.

"GFR is chemistry, bladder spasms are a plumbing problem", I tell her every time. "They are not related."

"I don't want to end up on dialysis and I have read that people with kidney disease are more likely to have heart attacks. My nephrologist tells me that, too. Mrs. Perlman said last Tuesday. Between her quarterly visits with Harold Wesson, the Chief of nephrology at Cityside Hospital, she worries enough to always mention her kidneys when she sees me for other things.

"But, Doctor, I have Stage III kidney disease!" Mrs. Jones said with obvious fear in her voice. It was Thursday afternoon and we really should have been talking about the dark mole on her right thigh.

"That doesn't mean you're in any real danger..." I began. She looked suspicious. "In fact, your kidney function two years ago was exactly the same."

"Are you telling me I had kidney disease already then?" Her eyes widened.

"To the same degree, yes. Do you remember how I asked you to stop taking ibuprofen for your sore knee because it could harm your kidneys?"

"Yes, that's when you gave me those prescription pain pills."

"Precisely. I was concerned then that we needed to be kind to your kidneys - that's pretty much all we do when people have what we call Stage III chronic kidney disease."

"But you never told me I have kidney disease."

"I didn't use the word because I feel it alarms people more than it helps them. We talked about what helps the kidneys and what hurts them; we got you off the ibuprofen, we tightened up your blood pressure control with a new medication and we lowered your cholesterol. All those things help your kidneys work better and last longer.

"But Stage III - I mean, how many stages are there? How close to dialysis am I with Stage III disease?"

I was ready for her question. With all the patients like her I have seen, especially lately, I have put together some articles and teaching materials.

"I have been a doctor since 1979 and I can count on one hand the patients I have cared for that ended up on dialysis or dying from kidney failure. Look at this graph", I said and pointed to the latest addition to my bulletin board. "You're 74, and your GFR is 54. This graph shows that at your age, your GFR would have to be somewhere around 15 to make you more likely to die from kidney failure than something else.

She stared at the graph.

"So 54 is actually not a bad GFR?"

"Well, it's not normal in terms of perfection, but it is very common. Even people who aren't perfect can live a long and happy life."

"So you're saying I shouldn't worry?"

"Not about your GFR specifically. Remember to be kind to your kidneys, like we have talked about."

She nodded.

"Now, here's the bad news", I explained. "People with even mild kidney disease statistically are more likely to have heart attacks, strokes and other cardiovascular problems."

She started to raise her eyebrows, and I hurried to continue:

"But, and this is important: I'm not smart enough to know what's the chicken and what's the egg. Do they have kidney disease because they have hardening of the arteries everywhere, or does the kidney disease itself cause it to happen?"

I continued:

"So we do the usual things - good diet, cholesterol, blood pressure. And we don't just focus on the GFR."

"I can't help worrying about the numbers", Mrs. Jones said.

"There's a name for that", I told her. "We call it albuminurophobia."

"Really?"

"Really. There is a medical term for just about everything these days."

She shook her head.

"Now, about this mole", I continued...

97) CHOLESTEROL GUIDELINES AND THE BACHELOR WITH PLATFORM SHOES

(This was my very first blog post on "A Country Doctor Writes, in 2008)

I have read that tall bachelors have more dates than short ones, and until recently it seemed obvious that men with low LDL cholesterol would have fewer heart attacks than men with higher levels. So what happens when a vertically challenged young man dons a pair of ABBA style platform shoes? And what does this really have to do with cholesterol?

Let me start from the beginning.

In medicine today, there are two mantras, even buzzwords: Evidence Based Medicine and Clinical Guidelines.

To practice Evidence Based Medicine is to do precisely those things that are proven by rigorous research to help the patient. Examples include giving heart attack survivors certain medications (Beta Blockers) or to give aspirin to patients with TIA's (often called "Ministrokes").

Clinical Guidelines often involve reaching numerical targets, and this is the first tip-off that we're on much shakier ground. Keeping a diabetic's blood pressure under 130/80 may be a good thing to do, but not if the person has a history of fainting from low blood pressure when standing up too quickly.

A dramatic example of failed guidelines came with the recent publication of the ENHANCE study (New England Journal of Medicine, April 3, 2008). The National Cholesterol Education Program has long recommended keeping the bad LDL Cholesterol under 70 in high risk patients, like those who have had a heart attack or a bypass procedure. The problem with this guideline was that it created a situation where doctors faced with an LDL slightly above "target" would abandon high doses of, for example the proven drug Lipitor, and switch patients to moderate doses of Vytorin, which contains a less powerful "statin" drug and an until now unproven new drug, called ezetimibe (Zetia).

The new drug, introduced in 2002, lowers cholesterol by blocking intestinal recycling of old cholesterol from the body's different cholesterol-based hormones etc. In the beginning, there was no proof that ezetimibe lowered heart attack rates or limited cholesterol buildup in our arteries, but there was something very promising about the drug; it not only helped lower cholesterol, but it also reduced levels of CRP, or C-reactive protein, an inflammation marker that closely follows heart attack risk.

So the number crunchers started to put pressure on doctors to reach numerical targets, and television ads promoted the dual action of Vytorin.

Fast forward to a couple of months ago when, after a billion dollars in sales, the new drug looks no better than platform shoes; better measurements, but same number of dates (in this case meeting our maker...), so to speak. The ENHANCE study didn't count deaths or heart attacks, but it did measure thickness of cholesterol buildup in arteries, and there was no difference between plain Zocor (simvastatin) and the combination drug (Vytorin). Factor in that you can buy simvastatin for $4/month at some supermarket pharmacies, while Vytorin costs 2,500% more (yes, do the math; $100 divided by $4 times 100%!).

The lesson here is that the guideline writers failed to think about what evidence we had about how patients achieved their goal numbers, just like the guy in the ridiculous shoes only thought he was closer to eye level with the girl he was trying to impress.

98) TWENTY QUESTIONS

Adrian Bell didn't look dehydrated, but his diarrhea had come and gone for a week and a half when I saw him a few weeks ago.

"Is anyone else sick with the same thing?" I asked, beginning my usual line of questioning.

"No", answered Eleanor, his wife.

"Have you had any water to drink from a new or unknown source, or have you traveled away from home?"

"No", both answered in unison.

"Any new foods that only you ate or that you don't normally eat? Are you a big milk drinker?" I added, thinking about secondary lactose intolerance.

Still, negative answers.

"Any chills, fever, belly pain..." my questioning continued.

Nothing.

"Have you had any antibiotics prescribed by any other doctor?" I asked, because we have had a flurry of Clostridium Difficile infections in our community, which is something we didn't have to worry about years ago. We had three cases recently at the nursing home, where Eleanor volunteers.

Still, "no".

"Anything else going on, even if it seems unrelated?" I finished my questioning as I motioned for Adrian to get up on the exam table.

"I have had some joint pains", he answered.

After an unremarkable physical exam, I ordered some lab tests, including inflammatory markers, a stool culture and C. Difficile test. I gave dietary instructions and we set up a follow-up appointment for a few days later.

At his follow-up visit, everything was the same and all the tests were normal. I sighed internally.

"Do you think it may be Beaver Fever?" Adrian and Eleanor both leaned towards me. "We've heard of an awful lot of people downstate who've had that."

"I haven't seen a case of giardiasis around here in years. How do you think you may have gotten that?"

"Well, two weeks before this started, I fell in a beaver pond in the woods in back of our property. I was checking out an old four wheeler trail...."

"Fell in a beaver pond..." I kicked myself for not having ordered a test for ova and parasites right away, but, of course, they can be unreliable.

"I think we've got to put you on some medication and do another stool test", I said, thinking to myself that I now have one more question for future diarrhea assessments.

Medicine is like twenty questions sometimes. If you don't ask the right questions, you don't get the right answers.

99) A TERMINAL CASE

When 87-year old Hildegard Mott was discharged from the hospital for the last time she was given less than six months to live. Her aortic stenosis was severe enough to cause chest pain at the slightest exertion, yet if she took nitroglycerin she invariably passed out. Sometimes she would pass out even without taking nitro.

She was given a prescription for liquid morphine to take if her chest pain became unbearable and Hospice nurses started to visit her a couple of times a week in her modest but spotless trailer in the Rainbow Hills trailer park just outside town.

The hardest part about coming home was that Sumner, her husband, friend and soul mate, wasn't there. He had died from a stroke just before Hildegard ended up in the hospital.

My house calls were special for both of us. She treated me like a son and never failed to tell me about her Scandinavian grandparents. Her own two sons live far away and I live an ocean away from my own mother. She told me of her symptoms and her worries. She knew her remaining days were limited; I had to certify a number less than the cutoff for Hospice services. Ironically, it was the hospitalists' idea to sign her up for Hospice, but I ended up certifying her prognosis.

She often spoke of Sumner in present tense. "I know he is here", she often said. "He comforts me when I am sad and calms me when my anxiety builds up. He helps me remember where I put things."

She seemed to hold her own as far as her symptoms went, but her days were long and her nights were lonely.

"I don't know why I am still alive", she would say. "If God wants me, I'd be happy to go."

"He must still have plans for you here", was my usual reply.

Many months went by and Hildegard had very little chest pain. She almost never took morphine and she seemed to know exactly how to pace herself. She always looked for the bright spots in everything that happened and lived her life in one-day increments.

Hospice finally terminated her case and she saw fewer interruptions in her solitude. She was weaker, there was no question about that, even though the more dramatic manifestations of her condition were less noticeable. She decided to look for placement in a nursing home.

That was four years ago. Hildegard settled in quickly at Leisure Ledges, and I visited her there now and then. Her favorite visits were the ones when I brought samplings of traditional Swedish foods. She always had visitors in her room because of her positive demeanor and kind interest in others.

Last Saturday night, almost five years after the hospital doctors pronounced her terminal, 92-year old Hildegard died in her sleep.

100) THE GIFT OF ONE DAY

A hard frost had claimed the white Geraniums in the flower boxes on the south side of the little red farmhouse a week earlier. Then Columbus Day weekend brought bright sun and the gift of summer temperatures again.

His family brought him outside around noon and placed him carefully near the east-facing wall where the unseasonable warmth of the sun and the gentle breeze made the temperature just right for the ailing elder.

His cough, which had rattled his chest every few minutes day and night for the past several weeks, ceased in the warm afternoon air. His facial expression relaxed with the slowing of his respirations. His clear, brown eyes squinted in the bright light as his furrowed face turned toward the sun.

From where he sat he could see the tall apple tree in the front yard, the raspberry bushes by the edge of the woods, all leafless now, and the big asparagus patch in the middle of the east lawn. He knew every inch of this place; he could follow each path through the woods in his mind, even now when his legs couldn't carry him there anymore. He loved this place, this little farm, his place on Earth.

He fell into a quiet, blissful sleep. The neighbor's potato harvester groaned in the distance and the sound of restless geese, preparing for their autumn flight, echoed from the riverbank nearby. He nodded his head quietly without opening his eyes just as his favorite horse, a kind, gray mare, made her usual blowing sound of contentment from her sun drenched spot along the red barn wall. She stomped one hoof after the other into the hard barnyard ground to chase away flies that had returned with the warm weather.

Later, when Cindy and Adam pulled up the long driveway in their white convertible with the top down for the last time this season, on an impromptu foliage tour from the city, he opened his eyes and squinted in the sunlight again. He leaned forward and puckered his lips, half frowning, when their border collie lapped his scraggly chin like an ice cream cone.

Whenever Cindy and Adam came, it was always time for coffee. They offered him sips, but he didn't drink much. He fell asleep to the tinkling of cups and chatter of voices on the lawn as the warm afternoon inched toward evening and the sun moved westward across the sky.

He woke up with a slight chill and someone pulled his blankets tighter around his shoulders. He coughed slightly and the family quickly started moving inside.

He watched with a twinge of disappointment as Cindy and Adam piled into their little sports car and buckled the dog's harness in the back seat. They had a long drive back to town.

By suppertime he was fast asleep in his temporary bedroom in the glassed-in front porch with the heater going and several blankets to keep him warm. This space had allowed him to still be part of all the comings and goings of farm life while confined to his sickbed.

After the supper dishes were done and the barn animals had been tucked in for the night, everyone else went upstairs to their bedrooms. The old one slept peacefully in his glass bedroom downstairs under the cold, starry night sky. Frost formed again on the lawn and rooftops.

The goats chewed their hay. The gray mare stomped her hooves now and then against the barn floor. The old one's breathing grew labored and quick with a faint wheeze. A chevron of geese appeared in the southwestern sky. Their faint, rhythmic whooshing sound followed the breaths of the old one and grew louder as the birds' silhouettes crossed the bright yellow harvest moon on their long, inevitable journey from this one to their other home, thousands of miles away. As the sound of their flight grew quieter again, the respirations of the old one grew fainter and further apart. He was already almost home.

(For S...)

ABOUT THE AUTHOR

Hans Duvefelt received his medical degree at Uppsala University in Sweden in 1979. He practices rural Family Medicine in northernmost Maine. From age four, he knew he was going to be a doctor. Since 2008 he has written extensively about medicine and doctoring on his own blog and other sites including The Health Care Blog, KevinMD, Doximity, Australian Doctor, Medical Republic, Medical Observer, MedPage Today and Sweden's Allmän Medicin.